CUTE POODLES, SWEET OLD LADIES, AND HUGS

Cute Poodles, Sweet Old Ladies, and Hugs

Veterinary Tales

By

P.J. Miller, B.V.M.&S., M.R.C.V.S.

Published by thirty8street Publishing

ISBN Number 978-0692902806

Cover design by WordSugar Designs

Dedicated to my family, my staff, and, of course,

Newman (the best bulldog, ever)

Contents

Nobody Wants to Be a Veterinarian on Monday

Every Monday morning there is always one appointment that reminds you that it's Monday. Monday morning is never easy and straightforward. You can't hide from this either. Trust me on this one: I've tried. I tried booking time off and coming back on Tuesday or even Wednesday, and *it* will find you. Your first day back that morning will be your new Monday. I came to terms with this a long time ago. Some of my (least) favorite cases have started on Monday. This Monday was no exception.

I looked at the appointment schedule and already saw the signs. With computerized appointments, the appointments come with little notes or stories from the receptionist, giving information about the appointment. Back when old Grandpa was a veterinarian, they had an actual appointment book. The appointments were all handwritten next to printed time slots. They only had room for the owner's and the patient's name. They may have had a little note written in the margin somewhere. On rare occasions, they might have even used a Post-it note to remind some staff member about something that had to do with the appointment. When Grandpa was a veterinarian, it was either a lot simpler, or they had a lot of surprises.

Today our appointments come with a whole story attached. Sure, we get lucky sometimes, like when you just see "annual" that just means a yearly exam and vaccines. Another good one is "recheck." Those appointments don't happen all the time. No, what usually happens is, there is a story attached. Maybe biography is a better word, like, "Hasn't been to the vet in four years," "Owner says can be vicious, so use a muzzle," and another classic, "Owner can't be there. They're sending neighbor with the dog. Call them after you do your exam." The neighbor never knows anything about the pet, and then I end up playing phone tag with the actual owner all day. Even the simplest cases that roll in with the neighbor become a chore. If there is a lot of extra info, it's not going to be good news.

It was scheduled for 10:00 a.m. The name said it all, Anne Sweet. The staff had a nickname for Mrs. Sweet. It was "Mrs. Sweet-and-Sour." She got this nickname because of her extreme mood swings. Every time a staff member got off the phone with her or she left the practice, they would say either "sweet" or "sour," and you would know exactly which version they got. Usually we get served the sour version.

Mrs. Sweet was in her early seventies, and she had three small poodles. Like her, they had varying personalities. Betty and Ralph were nice and easy to deal with, but Cuddles was the complete opposite. She could be extremely vicious for a small poodle. One thing was for sure: she didn't like going to the vet and wanted no part of anything we needed to do. This appointment was for Cuddles. After all, it was Monday.

The appointment text said, "Vomiting all weekend. Diarrhea yesterday. Not eating. Owner can only come at 10:00." That last part is the receptionist's apology. She can only come at ten really means, "Look, Dr. Miller, I know it's Mrs. Sweet, it's Cuddles, and she is really sick. I know it's going to take a lot of time. I know all that. I tried, man! I really did. I swear. But you know Mrs. Sweet. There was nothing I could do."

Mrs. Sweet arrived exactly at 9:15 a.m. Yeah, that's right, forty-five minutes before her actual appointment. We all know she knows what time her appointment is; she made it an hour ago. She also had a ten-minute talk (sour version) with the receptionist. The poor receptionist always gets an earful about something. It's impossible to get her off the phone, and it's difficult to get her to change course once she goes off topic. "Off the reservation" may be more accurate. Since Cuddles was coming in for an upset stomach, Mrs. Sweet thought it relevant to relate to the last time Mrs. Sweet herself had a bout of GI problems. She described it as being so bad that it was more convenient for her to spend most of the morning on the toilet rather than getting up and having to go back. Mrs. Sweet offered her words of wisdom, telling the receptionist that "when you get older, dear, you'll learn there are just some things you can't eat."

She knew her appointment was at ten, but she always came early. Actually, *arrive* is more accurate. I don't think Mrs. Sweet goes anywhere. She *arrives*. When she showed up, it was a major production. The first thing you noticed was her fancy shirt or sweater. I don't know where she found her gear, but every shirt or sweater had poodles incorporated in it in one way or another.

"Hello?" she yelled. For her hello wasn't a friendly greeting as with the rest of the world. It was more like a reprimand. With that one word, she was not only announcing her arrival, but asking why you didn't open the door and greet her personally. What could you possibly be doing that was more important than that?

She was loud too. Most people have a volume control, but Mrs. Sweet only had two settings—loud and way too loud. My staff always complained that I was a loud talker, but she had me beat. Now don't get all soft on me; it was not a hearing problem. This was what we call in the veterinary profession a "behavioral" problem. She was carrying Cuddles under her arm and brandishing her four-pronged cane with the other.

"I'm here! Cuddles just spit up again before we left," she announced way too loud to the entire hospital.

Spit up is the same as vomiting. They don't teach you that in vet school. You're welcome. Some owners, especially older ladies, like to use the term *spit up*. My theory on this phraseology is by downgrading vomit to spit up, it will make their pet less sick. I'm certain they use the term to help them cope with the fact that their pets are sick and throwing up all over the house. Pets don't spit up; they vomit. They can regurgitate, but you can learn all the finer points about the way things come out that aren't supposed to if you go to vet school.

After a painful discussion about the details of her weekend cleaning up "spit up" and diarrhea, she took a seat in the waiting room. Mrs.

Perkins who came only for a cat nail trim had to endure Mrs. Sweet's step-by-step procedure for cleaning her dog's vomit and diarrhea. I felt sorry for Mrs. Perkins. I was told Mrs. Sweet made her write down the names of her cleaning products. We owe Mrs. Perkins one. That went beyond taking one for the team. It's not easy keeping Mrs. Sweet occupied for thirty minutes. We know.

Mrs. Sweet arrived in the exam room at 9:55 a.m. Even though we were five minutes early, she forgave me for being late. She told me she understood because her appointment was an emergency. I'm not sure exactly what she understands. Except for that arguably sweet comment, she went full-on sour mode. Normally the vet tech goes in first to get the pet's weight and a history. Then the vet goes in after. A history is the important information about the pet, information like the signs the pet is having (*sign* is a term vets use for *symptom*), for example, how many times it vomited, had diarrhea, or if it's eating. You get the idea.

For Mrs. Sweet, I go in with the tech. We evolved to do this for many reasons. We know she likes to talk and give details, lots of details. Sometimes she gets off track and starts stories that don't even have to do with her sick pet. Then there are the questions, lots of questions. They are not concerned-pet-owner questions. They are let's-pretend-you're-back-at-vet-school-and-the-professor-is-examining-you type of questions. So we want to save time and avoid all that, twice. Also, despite some of the complaints or stories my staff might tell you, I'm a nice guy. Really, that's true. If you pressure them enough, they will admit it. Case in point, I'm not subjecting them to a Mrs. Sweet history twice, so let's go in together and get this over with.

What went on in that exam room wasn't pretty by any stretch of the imagination. I could give you the play-by-play of my answers to Mrs. Sweet's interrogation, but I won't. I'll spare you the painful details of that exam-room visit, but don't worry: I'll share all the highlights. First, the infamous poodle T-shirt was in full effect. It was two poodles sitting next to one another, one black and one white. The white one was wearing a bedazzled Christmas Santa hat along with a bedazzled collar. The black one just had a bedazzled collar. I don't know why the black poodle wasn't partaking in the Christmas spirit. I also can't tell you why Mrs. Sweet would choose this festive attire for June. When I asked Mrs. Sweet about the number of times Cuddles vomited, she was quick to correct me (yell at me) that Cuddles hadn't vomited at all; she'd just spit up. It was finally determined to be ten times.

Here is another thing that you have to be aware of as a vet. Sometimes getting information from owners about their pets isn't as easy as you think. In fact, it's difficult each and every time. Let's take Mrs. Sweet. I told you she said ten times. You probably think I asked her, "How many times did she spit up?" I even used the lingo. Then she would answer directly, "Ten," right? What actually happens is most owners go off on a whole other tangent. This isn't just Mrs. Sweet; this is almost everyone. It went down like this:

"How many times did Cuddles spit up?"

"Well, she vomited once on Saturday. No, wait, it was twice because after the second time my neighbor came over to take me to the early bird at the Golden Corral. She had just come back from taking Nancy to the ER. That was 5:00 p.m. I remember because she was late!"

I have no idea who Nancy or the neighbor is either. But knowing Mrs. Sweet, I'm thinking at five o'clock that neighbor was on time.

Anyway, getting a history can be tough, but it's important to get the facts. No matter how painful it is. Sometimes, no matter how many times you ask a certain question, you don't always get the answer. Sometimes the facts get left out, and (spoiler alert) that is what happened in this case. More on that later. To summarize, I was able to pry out that Cuddles had vomited ten times, had five bouts of diarrhea, hadn't eaten all weekend, and had been acting depressed.

Cuddles was sick; there was no doubt about that. During the whole exam, she only tried to bite me one time, and it was a weak attempt.

If she was well, there be no exam or any procedure of any kind without a muzzle. From her exam, I could tell her abdomen was painful.

The next steps were to do blood work and X-rays. The plan was to keep her in the hospital on IV fluids until we could figure out why she was sick, and treat her symptoms. I knew that plan from the beginning. Mrs. Sweet was a knowledgeable owner. She already knew it as well. She was a great owner who loved her dogs, and always did what I recommended. I knew she trusted me. Going over the plan with her, you wouldn't think so. If you were in that exam room with us, you would be thinking the exact opposite.

Every test, every treatment I recommended started a lengthy discussion. She was sure to bring up plenty of examples of dogs she owned with similar signs in the 1980s, dogs that were treated way back when by her old vet and his old-school voodoo medicine. Lastly, she wanted a breakdown of almost every what-if scenario. When it came to Mrs. Sweet, if you were a new vet on the job, you'd be in real trouble.

11:05 a.m.

Mrs. Sweet said goodbye to the receptionist (screamed, "I'm leaving! Tell Dr. Miller to call me later with an update!" to the entire hospital) and left. As she walked out, if you were sitting by the receptionist, you'd have heard the receptionist whisper, "Sour," just as the door closed.

Cuddles was a ten-year-old white toy poodle. For a female toy poodle, she was rather large. She was slightly overweight, but at seventeen pounds, she was way beyond the ten-pound toy poodle. Before we go any further, there is something important you need to know.

The general public (everyone who has never worked at a veterinary hospital) doesn't have a clue about what we go through. The popular fairy tale about working at a vet hospital is that we all get to play

12

with dogs and cats all day. People picture us treating cute pets, after which they lovingly lick our face while their owners tell us how great we are. I'm not going to lie: that can happen. Looking back, I think it's even happened to me about three, maybe four, times.

No, what we really go through every day is much different. The reason I bring this up, you're about to read a story about a seventeen-pound poodle named Cuddles. What could be so hard about that? The average person stops listening closely to that story after that sentence. No matter how hard you try and explain what went down, his or her mind is going back to that original fairy tale. They're thinking, "C'mon, man, it's a toy poodle owned by a lady who wears bedazzled shirts." Those of us in the veterinary trenches, we know better. We know what really goes down.

Getting a blood sample from her was no easy task. Whatever sick trance she was under before in the exam room had worn off. As soon as I pulled the cap off the syringe to get her blood sample, Cuddles decided it was go-time, and she let out a high-pitched, bloodcurdling bark. For good measure, she decided to have a large bout of foul-smelling diarrhea all over Cassey, the tech holding Cuddles. When she turned to bite Cassey's right cheek, I decided using a muzzle was definitely the way to go. Cassey is a pro, and was able to avoid getting bit, but not that nasty diarrhea. You can't dodge that bomb.

Don't worry. I know you're an animal lover. So am I. Cuddles wasn't extremely stressed or scared. Not this dog. Cuddles is aggressive, and she wants to be the boss. She wants to do what she wants, when she wants, and how she wants. She may be Mrs. Sweet's precious angel but not in our practice. Here is a fun fact: it has been scientifically proven that dogs are incapable of being spiteful. Even though I want to believe that diarrhea was meant for us, it wasn't. That fact is important to know when you hear owners who think their pet's accident is part of a secret plot to ruin their lives or get revenge. The bad news is that their pet is not housebroken, and the blame is all on the owner.

Ten minutes, a muzzle, and one scrub top later, we got Cuddles's blood work. We were also able to take X-rays of her abdomen. We got lucky for that ten minutes. Cuddles had exhausted herself temporarily, which made things go smoothly. The next step was to get an IV catheter in her leg and start her on fluids. Dogs and cats can get catheters in their legs and receive fluids just like people. The difference is when Nancy went to the ER from food poisoning and they put her on fluids, I'm fairly certain, she didn't react like Cuddles did. Yeah, that's right. I heard the whole Nancy story from Mrs. Sweet later that week. It was in the middle of talking about Cuddles and had absolutely nothing to do with what I was explaining to her. Mrs. Sweet would want you to know the good news is Nancy is fine, but more importantly, it wasn't the Golden Corral.

Most pets are OK about getting an IV catheter placed, especially taking into account that you can't explain things to them as you would a person. It does help to have a calm, reassuring tone and work slowly, but beyond that it's roll the dice. Sometimes we like to think we'll get lucky. What this means in medical terms is I like to try if I can do simple, nonpainful procedures without sedation. The techs don't always see eye to eye with this philosophy. Sometimes, it seems like they want to sedate everything. This might have to do with the fact that they always anticipate the worst and want to make their jobs as easy as possible.

We started with a muzzle and a lot of the calm-and-go-slow technique. We got her leg shaved and cleaned without any struggle. With Cassey holding, Jen, our head tech, got the IV catheter in. The last part is to tape it in so it stays in place. As Jen reached for the tape, I told them I was right about that whole no-sedation thing. Just then Cuddles decided our time was up. She bucked backward and then forward. In the process, she shook her leg from Cassey's hand and flung her catheter across the room on to the floor.

Even though nothing was happening to Cuddles at that moment, she decided to let out a high-pitched bark that sounded more like a scream. I'm pretty sure every client in the building heard it and was wondering whose dog was getting abused. Thanks, Cuddles. If that wasn't enough, she decided it was a good time for another episode of nasty diarrhea.

Good news, Cassey and her scrub top were spared. What wasn't good is that it was twice as much as last time. Cuddles decided to back up into it, and then use her hind legs to fling it all over the treatment area. She then relaxed, calmly squatted on the table, and urinated. After, she cocked her head to the side and licked her front lip through the muzzle. It appeared she was trying to convey some sort of message. I don't know what the message was, but we could definitely see and smell it. It was the most relaxed I had seen her all morning. Once everything got cleaned up, including me, the second catheter attempt went great. I forgot, on purpose, to tell you that my cheek got hit by the last storm out of Cuddles. With Cuddles resting in a cage and on IV fluids, I had a chance to look at her results.

First up was her blood work, known in veterinary circles as her *superchem* and *CBC*. Without taking you through the last three years of vet school, basically the superchem tells us about how well her internal organs are functioning. The CBC looks at her red and white blood cells. More importantly the white-cell part of the CBC can tell us if she has an infection. Cuddles's superchem was normal. Her CBC showed she was mildly dehydrated (from the vomiting, diarrhea). Her WBC was normal.

On her X-rays, I was looking to make sure she didn't have a blockage, for example, if she'd eaten something she shouldn't have, like one of her toys, a rock, or her owner's sock. I also wanted to make sure there wasn't anything in her abdomen like a tumor. Her X-rays were also normal. I didn't have an answer to why she was vomiting and having diarrhea. I had a good guess, though.

There was one test that I wouldn't get the results on until the next day. It was another blood test, and it had to be sent to an outside lab. It was a specific test for the pancreas. As in people, it sits at the base of the stomach. One of its jobs is to digest fat. If it gets inflamed or irritated (pancreatitis), it can cause vomiting and diarrhea.

15

"Slow down, Doctor! You speak so fast I have no idea what you're talking about!" I'd just finished my last appointment of the morning, and I was on the phone with Mrs. Sweet.

"I said, everything looks good so far, and we are waiting for her pancreatitis test to come back tomorrow morning. She hasn't had any more vomiting, but she has had two more bouts of diarrhea. She's a little dehydrated. With all the vomiting and diarrhea, I think she needs to stay here overnight on fluids."

"You keep talking about vomiting! She never vomited. She only spit up! You have to slow down I don't understand this *pan-krea-titas* thing you keep saying, or how she'd even get that! What time should I come get her this afternoon?"

"Mrs. Sweet, she's pretty sick. I think you should keep her here overnight, so we can keep her on fluids—"

"Wait!" she interrupted me. "You know what? I have a better idea. I think you should keep her. I think you should keep her on fluids there overnight! I don't think I should take her home this afternoon. That's what my vet up north did with my poodle Bo-jangles. He told me he slept in the cage with him all night to keep him company." I'll spare you the rest of that story. "What about this pan-kre-atis. How'd she get that? Can my other dogs get that?"

"No, Mrs. Sweet, it isn't contagious. The most common way they get it is from table food, like steak, fried food, or eggs—"

"I don't know how many times I have to tell you, Doctor. I don't give my dogs table food! I told you that already this morning. You keep going on and on about that. So how'd she get this *pan-krea-isis*? And how are we going to treat it!"

"I don't know that she has that yet. I need to see the test results tomorrow."

"Well, what's wrong with her then?"

"Right now, we are treating her for an upset stomach. She is on fluids, and I'm going to start her on some medicine for her diarrhea."

"Upset stomach! *Pan-kri-titass*? I'm confused now. Too many details. I have to get my hair done, and I'm late now, because I was waiting for your call all morning! Call me later, and let me know how she's doing. Hopefully, you can figure out what's wrong with my girl. I know you will take good care of my baby. Goodbye, Doctor. I have to go!" Click. She did say one nice thing. I always try to focus on the positive, but it rarely works for me.

By the afternoon, Cuddles was starting to improve and act more like herself. Randomly, she'd pick on patients we brought back to weigh and start aggressively barking at them. It didn't matter if the dog was four times her size. Through the bars of her hospital cage, she'd have a go at them. Her cage was at the back of our treatment area, and she was in the top row, four feet from the floor. It didn't matter how far away she was, she owned the entire treatment area. The other dogs would look back and ignore her, realizing she was in a cage and confused why a small dog would act that way. Unaware of what we call *little-dog syndrome*.

It's not a real syndrome or condition. Little-dog syndrome is when small dogs act aggressively to other dogs, especially large dogs. There are a lot of factors involved in this, including how they are raised by their owners. And there may also be a genetic component to this personality. Unfortunately, it can get these dogs into trouble. It has led to a lot of stitches at my practice. I had one more appointment before it was time for the last Mrs. Sweet update of the day. It wasn't an easy one as I'd thought either.

The appointment just said, "Annual and vaccines." You know what I was thinking—quick exam on a healthy dog and vaccines, simple. Then call Mrs. Sweet and this Monday would be over. The appointment was for "Gina," a four-year-old dachshund. After the techs got done getting her history, yearly samples, and weight, I grabbed her chart. The first thing that caught my attention was her weight. Last year her weight was sixteen pounds. Her weight today was twenty-two pounds. I asked Jen to get her out and weigh her again. Knowing Jen, I instantly knew how that request would go over.

"I don't know why you always do this, Dr. Miller. The scale isn't broken. When you see Gina, you'll see it's right," she grumbled. I had to double-check it. It's part of being a good doctor. It's never fun doing something simple twice, and Jen never lets me forget that either.

"See? Twenty-two pounds. I told you. You do this every time," she grumbled under her breath as she carried Gina back into the exam room.

"Hello, Mrs. Wilson, how are we doing today?"

"Busy. My daughter is away, and I have the grandkids."

Sitting on the exam room bench was a boy. He looked about ten years old. He was in shorts and T-shirt, glued to an iPad. Then a little girl, I'm guessing four years old, jumped out from under the exam room table and yelled, "Boo! I gotcha, Dr. Muller!"

Yeah, you got me, kid. It's Miller, though. Gina was on the floor now. The little girl had got her all excited. Gina was doing laps around the exam room, jumping off and on the bench and barking. None of this fazed the boy on the iPad; he didn't move.

"Lily, stop it and sit next to Alan!" Mrs. Wilson exclaimed. Mrs. Wilson was a tall, skinny woman in her seventies. She could pass for younger, even with her long, gray hair. She was a great client and pleasant to deal with. Jen bent down to pick up Gina and put her on the exam table. I was finishing my exam when Mrs. Wilson started.

"I know what you are going to say. Gina is fat." She was right, except I try not to use the *fat* word. I'll admit I'm known by my staff and clients as being straightforward and to the point. Sometimes being straightforward is good. Sometimes it's not. I have been on both sides of this fence, trust me. My staff would be quick to tell you I've been on that wrong side a lot, too often to be exact.

18

"Yeah, you beat me to it, Mrs. Wilson. I'd say she has gained a lot of weight in a year. She went from sixteen to twenty-two pounds. That's a big difference," I said, finishing my exam.

After I gave Gina her vaccines, Jen put her back down on the floor and quietly exited the room. *Disappeared* is probably a better word. In her defense, she was done helping me and why suffer through another Dr. Miller weight-loss talk? It was either that or she predicted the chaos that was about to transpire. Either way she was gone.

"I don't know how she got so fat. I feed her the same amount every day. She hardly gets any treats."

"Does she get table food?"

"No, never. At least not from me. Maybe my husband. He never listens to me. Maybe the kids slip her stuff when they stay with me," she whispered (poorly).

"No, we don't, Grandma! Dr. Miller, Grandma takes Gina through the drive-through with us. Gina loves McDonald's hamburgers. Grandma always gets her one."

"Shhhhh, that's not true!" Mrs. Wilson said, gesturing to Lily to be quiet.

They are all guilty. I might let Alan slide. He's too busy on the iPad. What's more irresistible than cute little Gina? Well, she used to be little. It is rare for an owner to admit it's his or her fault. I think that has happened once in my exam room. It's always the spouse, the kids, anyone but them. If they aren't in the exam room that day, they're getting the blame. I have even seen them turn to the pet and ask, "Are you sneaking food behind my back?" Let's face it: the pet isn't feeding itself extra food or driving the car to the drive-through.

"It is OK, Mrs. Wilson. We are on your side. I'm not here to judge, trust me. I'm here to help you. We are on the same team." That's all true.

She got the whole talk, the one staff had heard more times than they could ever want. Like a lot of talks, they could recite it word for word on their own. It's part of the reason that when they get the chance to break out, they take it. Summary: Feed less. Measure her food. No table food. Especially, no table food! That's a big one. Aside from making dogs overweight, it's the most common cause of vomiting and diarrhea that we see. There is some table food that's OK, but it's definitely not McDonald's hamburgers. Dachshunds are prone to pancreatitis. I told her that too. If you're keeping score, it was the fourth time she got it in the last four years.

I was finishing up when it hit me. The smell. I hate to admit, but it's one I'm very familiar with. Yeah, it was dog shit. Apparently, it was time for Gina to go, and the exam room seemed as good a place as any.

"Grandma? Grandma! Gina poo-ed. Eeeeewwww! Nasty!" Thanks for the breaking news, kid. But wait: it gets better. "Grandma, Alan made me step in it! Sorry, Dr. Miller, I think I got some on the floor there." She pointed to one spot, but looking closely, it was a lot more than one.

I have to hand it to Alan, or whatever app he was on. Despite Gina going to the bathroom a foot in front of him, and then his sister accusing him of somehow being involved in this mess, he never moved. He might have groaned, but that was it.

"Oh, Lily!" Mrs. Wilson sighed. It was then Lily opened the exam-room door to go out into the hallway. I don't know what it is about that door. Little kids love it. More specifically, they love the doorknob. It never fails. It might appear to be an average doorknob, but to kids, it has a magical allure. They are drawn to it. During every appointment with small children, that door gets opened at least twice, usually at the worst times, case in point.

The other fascination is the light switch. I can't tell you how many times I've had to talk to owners in the middle of a child-induced, flickering light show.

"Lily, stay here!" Well, Lily did, but Gina, she's good. Really good. Don't let that chubby little body fool you. She was gone. She couldn't go anywhere but the hallway. Not to worry unless you're a tech. That's another "clean up on aisle two." Gina also stepped in *it* and dragged *it* up and down the hallway. I think that when she put her paws up on the front desk, there was also a spot. Mrs. Wilson took off Lily's shoes, and we gave her a plastic garbage bag. She apologized. She apologized a lot.

The staff got homemade chocolate chip cookies the next week, but that wasn't until a week later. My thanks to Mrs. Wilson; they were great. I ate more than my share of them.

So, with no clients left in the building, it was tech vent time. Yeah, it's not fun cleaning that up, and they had a rough day. I give them credit. A lot of credit. For now, it was time to complain. I heard all about Cuddles, Mrs. Sweet, catheters, diarrhea, and ground-in dog shit. I even got yelled at for pointing out the stuff by the counter. I also heard something about me talking too long. I think I heard that twice. Face it: we both know I'm as guilty in this as Alan was. I let them vent. They deserve it. Without a great staff, you'd be nothing. I don't care how great a veterinarian you are—without a great staff behind you, you'd be in trouble.

I called Mrs. Sweet. "Hello, Doctor. I knew it would be you. How is my Cuddles doing?" I don't know if she has caller ID, but at 5:10, she had a good shot of answering the phone that way and being right.

"Pretty good actually. No diarrhea since we spoke last, and we are going to offer her some food."

"What kind of food? Do you know what she likes? She is real particular!"

"It's a bland diet that we have here. It allows her digestive system to rest."

"By the way I found an old copy of *Reader's Digest* from 1998 laying around, and it talks about *pancree-et-tis*. It says it can be caused by gallstones. Did you look for those? Does Cuddles have gallstones!" Since Mrs. Sweet doesn't have the Internet, you'd think I'd get a pass on these types of discussions. But whether it's her neighbor, *Reader's Digest*, or one of her previous medical experiences, I still get nailed.

"No, Mrs. Sweet, it's not gallstones. Dogs are different than people. Large gallstones show up on X-ray. Gallstones that cause a blockage would have shown elevated liver values in her blood work. I don't think she would be acting this bright if she had a blocked gall bladder."

"Slow down, Doctor. None of that makes any sense. You know I'm not a doctor. I do know poodles, though, and have had them for many years. Did I tell you my vet up north told me I should have been a vet? I have an instinct about these things, Doctor. You may want to look into the gallstones. Luckily, I found that *Reader's Digest*. I can bring it to you tomorrow if you want."

"No, Mrs. Sweet, that's OK. How about we wait for the pancreas test first? We are going to offer her the bland diet. She'll stay on the IV fluids for now. Jen will come back and check on her tonight and call you with an update."

"What time? You know I go to bed early!"

"Jen usually comes in around 10:00 or so—"

"Tell her if Cuddles is OK she doesn't need to call me. Doctor, when you get to be my age, sleep is precious. I was up all night worrying about Cuddles, and I slept on the couch. That couch is so old it's hard to sleep on it as it is. It's not like my bed. I almost fell asleep getting my hair done. I'm tired! Plus, I have to go tell my neighbor how Cuddles is doing. She wanted an update. I have to go. Thank Jen for me. Call me first thing in the morning when you get the gallstone test back."

If I wanted to debate her last statement, she was gone before I could say goodbye. Finally, another Monday was finished.

Tuesday

I came in to find Cuddles exactly how I expected, barking up a storm. When Jen had called me on Monday night, it had been all good news. Cuddles had eaten all her food, no diarrhea or vomiting. Cuddles had also tried to bite Jen after her walk that morning. I grabbed the chart to check her PLI (pancreas) test. Normal is less than 200. Cuddles was at 795. Pancreatitis. In cases like this, it's always table food until proven otherwise. I picked up the phone to call Mrs. Sweet.

"Hello, Doctor, how's my girl? What'd the test say?"

"It says she has pancreatitis. Normal values are less than 200. Her test was 795."

"Slow down, slow down with all these numbers. I don't need the exact numbers. I'm not a doctor. She has the *pancree-atit-tis*. What about the gallstones? My neighbor told me her sister had gallstones. Sounded just like Cuddles."

"It's not gallstones. It's pancreatitis, inflammation of the pancreas."

"How she'd get that! Doctor, I don't understand!" She was starting to get frustrated.

"Mrs. Sweet, I want you to think carefully back to late last week. Anything she could have eaten that's not dog food?"

"No, she only gets dog food! That's all. Wait. Slow down. Hold on. Let me think a minute! I did go out for Chinese food on Friday for dinner. I brought home the leftovers. I usually have them the next day for lunch. Ralph and Betty were sleeping in the living room. Cuddles, she followed me to the kitchen and was giving me her look. I felt so bad, I gave her some noodles and vegetables. It was the smallest bit. That couldn't have done this. It was such a small amount, and that stuff is healthy."

Maybe to her this didn't qualify for the table food that I asked her about in the exam room. Sometimes getting facts from owners can be more of an interrogation, and once you have the hard evidence (results), they have no choice but to confess.

That's one I hear *a lot*. "It was just a small amount doctor. Just a morsel." It always is. Owners try to get themselves off the hook for giving their dogs upset stomachs. They'll think the smaller it is, the safer it must be. I'm not here to judge, but trust me: whatever they gave, it was more than enough.

"Mrs. Sweet, they stir-fry that stuff. It has a ton of grease. Greasy foods like that can definitely cause pancreatitis."

"I don't think that did it. It couldn't have been that. Just so you know, I also gave her a small piece of spring roll. It was just a taste. It does have pork, but I gave her mostly the vegetables. She's had that before, though, and never got sick like this! Maybe a spit up or a little reflux, but never sick. I get reflux from Chinese food too." Translation: *It always makes her vomit, but it's never serious enough to call you.*

"Well, Mrs. Sweet, you got lucky those other times. Kind of like driving a car without a seat belt, it only takes one time, right? Same with feeding your dog table food."

"I guess you *could* be right. Maybe they cooked it wrong, or she had a bad piece. Is she going to be OK?"

"She is doing great. As long she does well today, you can pick her up this evening."

"It has to be four thirty. I have dinner plans that I cannot miss!"

"Four thirty will be fine. If anything changes with Cuddles, we will call you."

"Thank you, Doctor, I will see you then," she said, morphing to the sweet version as she hung up the phone.

By the time 4:05 arrived, so had Mrs. Sweet. Brandishing her four-pronged cane, she exclaimed, "I'm here to pick up Cuddles. How are you doing, Liz!" She asked the last way too loudly to the receptionist.

"I'm doing great, Mrs. Sweet. Cuddles is definitely ready to go home." Mrs. Sweet thought Liz was referring to how much she missed her mommy, which she was. But Liz was also referring to the last thirty-six hours of having Cuddles hospitalized. The techs enjoyed not having to see Cuddles again until her annual, ten months later.

I stepped into the exam room to find Mrs. Sweet sitting down on the bench, smiling. "So, Doctor, is she ready to go home?"

"Yes, Jen will be in with her in a second." I went over Cuddles' aftercare: the bland diet for a week and the medication for the diarrhea. I slipped in another reminder about no table food. Only time and the medical records would tell if and how long the promise she gave me would last. I'm not that optimistic. Hearing "undercooked," "bad piece," and "I gave her too much" tells me she'll be back again.

Jen came in with Cuddles. Cuddles pulled to the end of the leash until she jumped up into Mrs. Sweet's arms. Cuddles then started licking Mrs. Sweet's face as if they had been apart for years. You would have thought it was another dog that we had hospitalized. I'm not going to lie: that thirty seconds right there is the best part of my job. It was then that I realized Mrs. Sweet was wearing a plain, white V-neck T-shirt with a bedazzled collar, but no poodles. What? No poodles?

She stood up thanking me profusely. I think a hug might have actually been involved. Anytime the techs catch wind of something like that, I get harassed for a week. The hug, maybe I'm not remembering that last part right. I do remember catching a glimpse of her pants as she walked out of the exam room with Cuddles under her arm. They were light-blue cotton pants with tiny white poodles

25

printed over them. I also remember the one word that came to mind as I left the exam room: **Sweet**.

Fallback Career

It wasn't my original plan to be a vet at all. Really, that's true. This is not how it was supposed to go. Even my fallback career path was going to be different than what went down in chapter 1. In fact, if things had gone the way I'd initially planned, I wouldn't have become a veterinarian. No chance. When I was younger, my plan had been much different.

I was born and raised in Midtown Manhattan. Growing up, basketball was my life. I played it every chance I got. Indoor gym or outside on the street court, it didn't matter. In New York City, there was a good chance there was a game going on some court somewhere. On the off chance there wasn't, I shot baskets on my own. I'd even shoot around in the snow. My initial plan—dream is probably more accurate—had been to play in the NBA. Based on their inability to mentally conceive of me in any athletic-type role, my staff still laughs, no matter how many times I tell that story.

I don't know the exact date, but somewhere around the beginning of high school, that plan wasn't looking too good. I could see my height and lack of talent required to play at that level might be potential problems. I started to realize the NBA, fame, millions of dollars, and possible endorsement deals were not going to happen. It was then when I came up with my fallback career. It was solid! Now that could *actually* happen.

I was going to be a veterinarian! It was not going to be like that sucker in chapter 1. Not even close. That's way too much work and aggravation. No, I had it all figured out. I'd move to Los Angeles—more specifically, Beverly Hills. That's where you want a vet practice. I'm not dumb. That's where all the rich people live. I'm cool. I'm from New York City. They'd love me! I'd probably even have a few celebrities as clients. Even if they sent their assistants or relatives, I'd still be taking care of celebrity pets. Hey, who knows? I might even get famous myself. How hard could that be? That's the way to go. "Trim the nails on Buddy? No problem, you got it! Tell Brad (Pitt) Dr. Miller said what's up."

From a young age, I have always had a love of animals. Growing up, I had a lot of different pets—dogs, tropical fish, birds, and even lizards. The dogs were our family's pets. We always had at least one toy poodle. When I was six, we had the record of three of them. Yes, Mrs. Sweet was really happy when I told her that piece of family history. No, they weren't my choice. I loved all our dogs, but let's face: it's hard to get street cred with your friends, owning poodles. "Yeah, man, well, I got poodles," or "You don't want to break into my house, bro. My poodles will hear you coming from a mile away!"

I begged and pleaded with my dad to get me a "real dog." This went on for many years. It started in seventh grade. I bought a copy of the American Kennel Club book of dog breeds. It was a big, thick book, and every registered dog breed was in it. This way I could pick the perfect dog. I researched and showed him all the cool breeds. Bulldog? No! They drool, and your mom hates them. Boxer? No! Too big for an apartment! Bull terrier? You know, Dad—Spuds Mackenzie (the mascot for Bud Light in the '80s)? That one got a three-second pause. Even Dad knew that dog was cool, but still no! Well, you get the idea. In high school, I finally gave up.

There was more to that story than my dad just not wanting to walk another dog or have another mouth to feed. My brother had allergies and asthma. The only breed my brother could reasonably live with was poodles, because they didn't shed. On occasion, if he played with our dogs long enough, he'd start sneezing and have to take a Benadryl.

The other part of that story was it was my mother's favorite breed. After she'd moved to New York in her twenties, she'd always had at least one. In fact, she'd bred them once and had a litter. Don't tell my mom, but trust me: I'm glad I wasn't her vet for that one. My mom is not what I would call the ideal client. Whenever I talk about dogs with my family, they are all experts. Rather than defer to my opinion, it's always a discussion. There always the chance that they may know something I didn't. In fact, recently, my mom called me when I was on my way home from work. She told me she read an article in the newspaper that dogs can get diabetes, just like people.

"Did you know dogs can get diabetes? You should look into that."

"Yes, Mom, I actually do know that." I always joke that my mom is the veterinary chief of staff. My wife is the head resident, and I'm just the lowly intern.

My mom had kept one poodle from that infamous one-time litter. It would be the first dog I grew up with. He had been the runt of the litter, and no one had wanted him, so my mom had kept him. His parents, Frosty and Gigi, had passed away before I'd been born. He'd been the only black poodle we'd ever had. My mom had named him Baby. My dad thought that name was dumb, especially for a male dog, not manly enough. It was bad enough having poodles, but to have one named Baby? No, my dad wanted to name him Tarzan. What's more manly than the king of the jungle? Now that's a man's name! Well, they never agreed on his name. My mom always called him Baby, and my dad always called him Tarzan. So, he was known as Baby, Tarzan, or Baby-Tarzan. He'd come to all three. I called him Baby. He was an awesome dog. Despite his name, being the runt, and supposedly a toy poodle, he was huge. He weighed roughly twenty pounds.

As a toddler, I'd never left him alone. He'd been my best friend. I'm sure that to him at times I had been more like his frenemy. No matter what I'd poked, prodded, or pulled on him, he never bit me. Not once. He played his part, or character, in whatever game we were (I was) playing, and without complaint, even if that game had meant being a horse. I can remember the time I stood over his back. I'd held his collar and walked him around the apartment like he was a horse. Well, maybe it was more than once. He never protested, barked, or cried. He would play along, kiss me, and follow me when it was over.

29

When I was five, we got two more poodles, a brown male and a white female. The male was named Napoleon. I asked my dad about his name when I was older. He told me, "It implied he might be small, but he doesn't take anyone's shit! Just like Napoleon."

The female, Gigi, I don't know what it was with my mom and white female poodles named Gigi. Everyone she had would be named Gigi. This was the second Gigi, or she would sometimes affectionately say "Gigi the Second." It was as if they were poodle royalty. We would go on to have three Gigis. The third was my favorite.

Napoleon was around twelve pounds. He had an outgoing personality, and was friendly to everyone. He would be the first dog that my dad would try and "train" to be an "attack dog" (if you want to call a poodle that). Every time someone came to the door and rang the bell, my dad would get the dogs all worked up. "Who's there? Who's that! Get 'em! Sick 'em! Bad man! Sick him!"

Napoleon would act ferocious, but he never bit anyone. He would snap at people coming to visit but fell short of any real contact. Gigi II was a tiny dog from the start. I don't ever think she made it past five pounds. She was always very weak and frail and not very active as far back as I could remember. Because of these genetic limitations, she was never accepted to Miller's attack dog school. As you can already tell, none of these dogs got me any cool points when my friends came to visit. My mother blamed it on the anesthesia Gigi had when she was spayed. It was with our first vet in New York City, who I never met. "She was never right after that. It was that *anesthee-gia* (in her German accent). That's what did it."

To this day, I don't really know why Gigi II was like that. Anesthesia, even back then, is pretty much an all-or-nothing deal. Either you make it or the other outcome (we won't mention) that rarely happens. Today, I quote that outcome at less than one percent. I'm not a big fan of the older generation of veterinarians (if you haven't already guessed), but this vet had a great reputation. It was well deserved. I never believed the anesthesia answer, even after vet school. After Gigi (the second) and Napoleon were gone, we got the last Gigi.

Gigi the Third was different. We got her when I was fourteen. As a kid, she was the first real dog we ever had. Her personality was extremely outgoing. She had a ton of energy. It was as if she never outgrew being a puppy. She was pretty stout for a female. She weighed in at about fifteen pounds. She loved everyone in our family. If you were in bed, she'd be there. All of our dogs slept in our parents' bed. As kids, we tried to put them in our bed, but they'd jump out. Not Gigi III. She was different. If anyone slept late or was sick in bed, that is where she'd be. Every time someone came home, it didn't matter if you were gone for hours or months, she would go ballistic. She'd be barking and jumping all over you.

If any dog were to graduate from Miller's attack dog school, it'd be her. She would graduate with honors. Anyone who came to visit, she would instantly attack and bite. In fact, she became a legend in our building and not in a good way.

My father was taking Gigi out to do her daily "bizness." They were riding the elevator in our building on the way down. When the doors opened on the eighth floor and Adele stepped in, that is when it all went down. Adele was a slightly (maybe more than slightly) overweight lady, who at the time was in her early sixties. She had short (dyed) blond hair, and small beady eyes. She always wore a muumuu dress and house slippers. Every day she was in the lobby of our building, gossiping and minding everyone else's business. For her, asking how people were doing was more of interrogation than a friendly conversation.

When Adele made her way into the elevator that day, Gigi ran to the end of her leash, leapt into the air, and attempted to bite Adele's hand. The bite was supposedly so bad that she sat in the lobby all day. She sat there, holding her hand and complaining to every person who came and went into our building. Most people who knew her habitually tuned her out. The others stopped listening after they heard "white poodle" and failed to see any bite marks on her hand.

31

The story still became legendary in our building, and she told people that she was going to sue my father. My father never liked Adele before, and after that incident he took great joy in messing with her. Every time he saw her sitting in the lobby, talking and not paying attention, he would surreptitiously start barking and growling like a dog. For the record, she never did pursue legal action or get any medical attention for her supposed dog bite.

There were times when Gigi did actually bite people. A lot of my friends, and even my wife will to this day still complain about getting bit by her. In high school, I'd hear, "Yeah, I went to his house. That dog bit the crap out of me, man! She's crazy, bro."

"You mean that little poodle. Isn't *her* name *Gigi*? Hahahaha, Gigi," they'd fire back to the victim. To which the victim would reply "OK. Wait till you go there, man. We'll see what you say then. Watch!" If a poodle could ever get you any kind of street cred with your friends, Gigi the Third would be the one to do it.

I was fortunate. I was always a good student all the way through to high school. I never really enjoyed school (who does), but if I had to pick a favorite subject, it was science. I graduated high school in the top ten percent of my class. I can't remember my SAT score, but trust me: it wasn't great. I never have done well on multiple-choice tests, more on that later. I had some great recommendations from my teachers, though, and with that, I was accepted to the University of Florida. It was actually my first choice.

Growing up, we spent two weeks almost every summer in South Florida. My father was from Brooklyn. My dad's side of the family moved to Hollywood, Florida, before I was born. I loved going down to see them. As a kid, I loved New York City, but the change and weather in Florida had me hooked from the start. Like all teenagers, at seventeen I was ready for that kind of change. I also thought that since UF had a veterinary school, I'd have a better chance of getting in as student of the university. FYI, that's only a little bit true.

When I first got to the University of Florida, I was definitely like a fish out of water. The majority of the students were from Florida. I was straight out of NYC, and it was obvious. My thick New York accent was a dead giveaway. Then, apparently, what's cool to wear in high school in New York isn't cutting it at UF. I might as well have been a foreign exchange student. For the first couple of months, I felt like one. I instantly gravitated to the students from the big cities like Miami. If they were from New York, even better. I felt their pain with these "country folks" and connected instantly. I'd had a preview of this culture shock before.

It had been when I'd come down for an orientation weekend with my father, months before school actually started. We flew into Jacksonville, rented a car, and drove to the University of Florida in Gainesville. My dad was lost. The temperature was in the nineties. We didn't have GPS or Siri to help us back then. When we arrived at a stop light next to a pickup truck, Dad rolled down the window and asked for directions.

"Can you tell me how to get to Gainesville?" he asked in his thick Brooklyn accent.

The man in the pickup truck replied in his country accent, "Gainesville? Gainesville! You in Gainesville, boy!" The driver let out a laugh as he drove off when the light changed. We were on the outskirts of town and hadn't even known it. What I also hadn't known was that was a dose of some of the country flavor I was about to get.

My major at UF was animal science. Animal sciences majors learn about the nutrition, breeding, behavior, and management of food animals (farm animals). Basically, with this major you are either applying to vet school or working in a job that has something to do with farm animals. In order to apply to vet school, you had to fulfill all the required pre-vet coursework; you didn't actually need a specific major. If you were a certified genius, you could take only the prerequisite classes in three years, apply, and get in. In my career, I have only met two veterinarians that did that and were able to get in.

I chose animal science because I wanted to get farm-animal experience. Being from NYC, I thought it would make me a more well-rounded applicant (look good on my resume). The only farm-animal experience I'd had had been when I visited my mother's family farm in Germany a few times when I was young. When I say farm, we're talking old school. It wasn't like the large-scale industrial farms that are common today. It was a small farm with some milking cows, a few pigs, and some chickens.

Animal science wasn't a fallback career either. I was getting into vet school. Any kind of farm-related job wasn't an option. Let's face it: no one in any kind of farm-related business is hiring or taking advice from someone raised in New York City. My advisor was Professor Bill Graves. He was one of the older professors in animal science. He was in his early sixties when I first met him. He was tall and thin, and wore glasses. His skin was dark and wrinkled from hours outside in the Florida sun. The way he talked and carried himself, he was all business. He instantly gave you the impression that this was not a person you want to mess with. Like a lot of students and faculty in animal science, he wore a cowboy hat, cowboy boots, plaid shirt, and the big ole belt buckle. He had been at UF for a long time, and he was well liked and respected by everyone. When I met him the first time, that's all I knew.

I remember sitting in his office for the first time. The only things going through my mind were "I'm dead. This guy knows I'm a city boy and using animal science just to get into vet school. This is going to suck. It will be a long four years dealing with this guy." Every second he sat there, silent, looking at whatever info was on his paperwork, to me felt like years. Really, it was painful.

I was wrong. "So you want to be a veterinarian? That's great. I'm glad you chose animal science. I think that was a good idea, son, to getchu some farm-animal experience," he said in his thick Georgia accent. He warmed up to me instantly. He went over my first schedule. He even told me about the time he went to "Neu Yolk Citee." That was it. I learned later that with animal science students and professors, it would go one of two ways—in or out. There was no middle ground. They either loved me, or they hated me. It was instant. As soon as they heard me speak and figured out where I was from, it was either I was their new best friend or their mortal enemy. I could never figure out why it went one way of the other. What I could figure out instantly is where I stood.

My classes were another culture shock. I actually thought I was somewhat smart when I got to UF. I had done well in high school, and they'd accepted me, right? Well, I was in for another jolt. The class sizes I started out with were brutal. I had classes with hundreds of students in them. My grades were all over the place. Every test was multiple choice, and they were designed to catch you out, especially in classes like calculus. I hated that class. I hated it each of the three times I took it! That's not a misprint; you read that right, *three* times.

For me it was a killer, or more like a dream killer. The class was cruel. You could have a whole problem 99 percent correct, but mess up that last step, done, game over. Flip a positive or negative sign, be off by one digit, they'd get you. They'd have that answer waiting for you at the end next to an A, B, C, D, or E. You'd think you were right; you checked it three times. It's right there. It's "A) -5." Right? *Psych!* You're wrong. It's "5"; you messed that sign up in the second-to-last step, dumbass. Zero points. All the work you did to get there, that's worthless unless you got the *exact* answer. All or nothing. I never was a natural at math. The B-minus (my worst grade until now) I'd gotten in precalculus in high school had probably been an indication of what was going to happen.

When complaining about this horror story, other students told me that calculus was a *weed-out class*. They'd explain that a weed-out class is meant to do just that, weed you out. So many students wanted to be doctors or engineers they needed some way to find the best and the brightest. I don't know if that was actually by design, but looking back, there was a lot of truth to that. You'd have to be a genius, I thought, to pull an A in this class.

Calculus wasn't the only class like this either. There were other weed-out classes, like chemistry 1–3, organic chemistry 1 and 2, biochemistry, and physics. There were more, but those are the ones that traumatized me enough to remember them. I always wondered (complain and complain some more) why you needed calculus and physics to become a veterinarian. I'd hear from college professors, "They teach you problem-solving skills. Physics is involved in physiology." Spoiler alert. Guess what? They were all wrong. I didn't use any calculus or physics equations to treat Mrs. Sweet's dog.

I am not going to sugarcoat it. My first term, in fact my whole time at UF, was not pretty. It was a struggle, or battle was probably a better way to describe it. I was in good company, most all my friends at UF were pre-med or engineering. One of my good friends and later roommate, Heath, was in the same boat. Heath was also from New York City. He'd grown up in Queens. He was six feet tall, and he had short, jet-black hair that was always spiked. With his spiked hair, serious demeanor and muscular build, he looked intimidating.

For those of us who knew him, he was the complete opposite. He was a genuinely nice person. He was an extremely loyal and trustworthy friend. I am still friends with him today. Heath was an electrical engineering major. Not only did he have a lot of the same weed-out classes, but he had even more physics and math classes. Classes like differential equations. Looking at his notes from that class was like looking at foreign language. I couldn't even follow the first line of those equations.

To hear him talk about his classes or his professors, he sounded like a boxer and not a college student. "I can see already this class is trying to beat me, wear me down, knock me down, and make me quit." Or "Tomorrow I'm going to war with differential equations. I'm hitting that with basically everything!" Or my favorite, "Professor Shepard thinks he's slick, but after he grades my test, it's going to be a smackdown." Heath wasn't violent, but he was motivated.

I didn't have any pre-vet students as friends. There is a reason for that. After my first semester at UF, I found out about the "Pre-Vet Club." They held meetings on a regular basis to discuss everything and anything related to vet school. In these meetings, they discussed "important" pre-vet club business like guest speakers and future events. They had social events, fundraising events, events at local animal shelters, events with vet school professors, and events with veterinarians. Any kind of event they could possible plan and have, they had it.

It was a structured club with a president, vice president, and secretary. In some classes, I'd hear things like, "You remember Sarah. Well, she got in! I guess being president of pre-vet club really helped." Or "Oh yeah, if they see pre-vet club on your application that helps. It helps a lot." After hearing this and being anxious to do whatever it took to get into vet school, I decided to check it out.

The theme of all the meetings was the same:

"What grade you get in that class? A? B? Oh, you'll never get in with a B in that."

"How many volunteer hours do you have? Oh, you'll never get in with that. That's not enough. Where'd you volunteer again? Oh, that's no good, no good at all."

"Alison had great grades, and she's still a working as a tech. This is going to be her third time applying. She graduated like three years ago. She's got no chance."

After hearing all that negativity, I knew I'd do whatever it took to get into vet school, but I learned I was going to do it without the pre-vet club.

Looking back, people like Heath and my other friends never really doubted that I'd go to vet school and become a vet. For them it was like a given. They'd say things that included, "When you get in to vet school…" or "When you're a vet…"

It was no Disney movie. There was plenty of complaining, and I had real doubts that I would ever make it. I can remember getting a bad grade or test score and telling Heath, "That's it. I'm done, bro. It's over. I have *no* chance of getting in."

He always replied, "You'll get in. Trust me: you *will* find a way. You will get in." The way he said it wasn't just as a friend trying to make you feel better. No, the way Heath said it was that it was a well-known, accepted fact. As if he knew something I didn't. Heath was right.

By the way, I did run into the former president of the pre-vet club almost ten years later at another vet hospital. I was there for a job interview for a vet position. I remembered her instantly. Clair had been the golden child of the pre-vet club when I was at UF. She had been the president for three years and a shoo-in for vet school. I'd never liked her back then. In ten years, she hadn't changed. Unfortunately, none of the technicians at her hospital liked her either. Just like pre-vet club, she was still an arrogant know-it-all. Except she wasn't a vet—she was a technician. Just like nursing in human medicine, vet techs are the backbone to the veterinary profession. It is a great profession. But for Clair, who'd proclaimed herself as a soon-to-be vet for years at UF, being a tech was a tremendous blow to her ego.

For Clair, things probably didn't go as she had planned. I can relate to that. It was never part of my plan to end up as a college dropout. I never did graduate from UF. That's not just some catchy chapter title for chapter four. It's true. I officially dropped out in the last term of my third year. It was the best decision I ever made.

College Dropout

I'd just started my third year at UF. If you wanted to place a bet on my chances of getting into vet school, the smart bet was *no chance!* My GPA was just over 3.0. A B-minus average was not very competitive. By not very competitive, I mean the application with 3.0 on it is going into the garbage can as soon as they review it. Most of the weed-out classes had dropped a bomb on my GPA. If they'd wanted to weed me out, it was working. As far as bombs were concerned, calculus was the nuclear option.

The first time I had the pleasure of taking calculus was in the first term in my first year. My first two test scores were so bad I had no chance of getting the minimum C required. Even if I'd gotten a perfect score on all the remaining tests, I still couldn't have gotten a C. I decided to *drop it*. Dropping a class removes it from your record, but you still have to pay for it. There was a deadline to drop a class, and the second test was it.

The second time I took calculus was in the next term. For this "fight," I had Heath in my corner. He was now my roommate, and I could always count on him for advice. "Don't worry, bro. I'm the man with math—you know that. We are going to go to war on this class! That teacher is going to wish you passed the first time. When you get done, he will feel the pain. Each time he grades your test, he will feel pain. Because you aren't going to be a weed-out chump!"

First, teachers in a class that size actually didn't grade anything. It was a color in the circle for the answer, and a computer read the score. As far as the teacher was concerned, in a class of hundreds, he had no clue who I was or how many times I was taking the class. Lastly, I'm fairly certain he wasn't going to be upset (or in pain) if I did well in his class. But this was how Heath approached some of his toughest classes. It was a Heath-versus-[insert contender class here] fight to the death! It worked for him. His GPA was 3.8 in one of the hardest majors at UF. I adopted his attitude toward calculus.

"I just don't understand this, bro. I worked with you. You know the work. I can't see how it happened." It was one of the few times I actually heard Heath sound defeated. I had just told him my final grade in *Calculus the Rematch*. It was a C-minus. Below the required C needed for the pre-vet requirement. What made it worse was my last test score was one-point shy of getting me a C in the class. Heath was visibly depressed the rest of the day. He was so depressed he almost had me beat. It was as if he had gotten that C-minus. The next day, though, Heath bounced back and had a new plan.

"*Yo!* Listen to me for a second. OK, you have to retake it and pay again for that sucker. They *might* see calculus twice on your transcript. That's if they are actually are paying attention."

Just hearing that depressed me all over again.

"Listen, though! You know this work. If you get A or even a B-plus, your GPA will be better than if you got a C the first time. They are not going through and looking at each class. No chance. Trust me: there is no way they look at all those applicants' class lists individually. Not happening, bro. This is a win!"

Yeah, that speech was a big stretch on trying to be positive and flip the situation around. But what choice did I have? If I didn't meet the requirement, I'd have no chance at vet school. After he delivered it a few times I was fully on board. I was ready for *Calculus III: The Revenge*!

The grades were in. "Why are you upset?! This is good news. The B is solid. You never have to see that class again. Done!" I don't think I ever felt more disappointed with a B. It wasn't the grade we had planned on. It felt like an F. My nightmare with calculus was over, but the scar it left on my GPA was permanent.

With my GPA in the toilet, I had been working hard in other areas to help my chances of getting into vet school. I had been volunteering at a local horse farm that took in abused, neglected, and retired horses. They had over eighty horses spread out on their tremendous property. I was there every Saturday like clockwork. I'd work there from eight in the morning until two in afternoon. Any farm work they needed help with, I would do. Most of the work involved feeding and grooming the horses. I heard about the farm from the pre-vet club. I had stopped going to meetings as a member. But once in a while I'd "unofficially" attend a meeting. I do this to gain any information that I thought might be useful. The pre-vet club only went to the horse farm as an "event" once a year.

I was also working with a veterinarian in Gainesville. I arranged my class schedule to have Thursdays free. This way, every Thursday I could spend the whole day working with Dr. Silver. Dr. Eric Silver had also gone to UF, but he went to vet school at Mississippi State. His major was also animal science. He also thought the pre-vet club sucked. He had been recommended to me by Professor Graves in my first year. It was one of the best recommendations I ever got.

Dr. Silver had just bought his practice from an older veterinarian whom I never met. He was in his late thirties. He was short and stocky. He had thinning black hair that he cut short to help make his pending baldness less obvious. He was from Georgia and a true country boy. He loved giving me a hard time about being from New York City. He would always joke with his clients (especially the ones from the country) and tell them things like, "He got his animal experience working on rats from the street." His other favorite was when hardened cowboys would come in with their big farm dogs. He'd tell them that I grew up with all poodles. We all (they) would always have a big laugh about it.

He was a great person and mentor. His grades were better than mine when he was a student, but they were far from perfect. He was a great source for advice. It is why I asked him if I should apply to the Atlantic Bridge Program.

It was at the beginning of my third year when I heard about the Atlantic Bridge Program. You sent all your recommendations and college transcripts and filled out an application. The Atlantic Bridge Program would take all that and present it to the six vet schools in

Britain (at the time). I got the info about the program from an unlikely source, my father.

My father was a financial advisor in New York. It seemed as if he knew everyone. He was always telling me stories about people from all walks of life and in every profession imaginable. When he first told me about the program, I was skeptical. I figured he had no idea what he was talking about. Who's the pre-vet student? Who's read and heard everything about vet school here? Me, that's who! If this was a *real* program, I'd have heard about it, right?

"That program is probably for applying to medical school, Dad. Not vet school," I said.

"Stop arguing about it and look into it! OK?" my father yelled at me on the phone. If I held the receiver away from my ear, you still could have heard him.

"OK. OK. Calm down. I'll look into, OK? I promise."

"Look into it. Call *the* guy and tell me what he says." With my dad, it was always "a guy," "*the* guy," or "those guys." In this case, he was referring to the individual running the program, the guy who was in charge, *the* guy. My dad taught me from a young age it's always better to talk the "boss." The higher up that you start, the better results you'll get.

I looked into it. *The* guy was Ryan Kelly. He wasn't a vet, but he ran the program. He was from Ireland. When he heard I was from New York City, we hit it off instantly. He told me all about family he had in Queens. He took an instant liking to me, but that didn't change the news I got.

"The good news is the requirements in Britain are different than in the US. With the course work you have completed and will be finishing, you can apply now. I have to be honest with you, though. Your GPA is below, *way below*, what I have seen them accept. I don't want you to get your hopes up. I will also tell you can apply again next year if you aren't accepted. It will not affect your chances applying twice. My advice would be to get three very *solid* recommendations. I'd also try to get some spectacular marks this term. They will be looking critically at your last marks, as those are the most recent."

I was already working on the recommendations: the horse farm and Dr. Silver. Check. I needed a third, and Mr. Kelly had mentioned one from a professor. With my low grades and huge class sizes, that was hard to come by. There was one class in which my luck was about to change.

Organic Chemistry I had a reputation of being tough. When I say tough, I mean this was coming from students who got really good grades in the earlier weed-out classes. Heath had another technique that he employed for his hard classes: "Sometimes when I go to war with these suckers (courses and professors), I have to take it directly to them. I'll go to their office every day if I have to. I will live in that damn office. I will be their new best friend. I will know the work better than they do! That professor will be happy when that term is over." What he was referring to was seeing professors during their open office hours. If students had questions about course work, you could sign up for a scheduled time, and they would help you. This is exactly the plan I employed on Dr. Nobler.

I had gotten my intel, that there were two organic chemistry teachers. Dr. Nobler was the one everyone wanted. The other was nicknamed 'Dr. McMean' after the McDonald's hamburger at the time, the "McLean." His name is self-explanatory, and his tests were known for being ridiculously difficult. I requested Dr. Nobler's class, and I got it. The luck didn't stop there. For reasons unknown, the class size was smaller than usual. The class only had forty students. It made it easier to ask questions in class and get regular office appointments. He was even calling on people by name.

Dr. Nobler was a great professor. I would say easily one of the best I ever had. He was short, soft spoken, and bald, with thick-rimmed black glasses. He was exactly what you'd expect a chemistry professor to look like. He was extremely patient. It was obvious he was passionate about chemistry, and he loved to teach. This made going to his office less of a chore. Going to a professor's office that is cranky, doesn't like you, and hates teaching is torture. Heath had one of those, so I know. Heath went anyway, and "crushed" the class. I studied hours upon hours for Organic Chemistry I. I was also a regular guest in Dr. Nobler's office.

"B-plus, how you like that, Heath!" That organic chemistry grade was the best weed-out class grade I ever got. It was also the best term I ever had. The celebration was short lived after Heath calculated my GPA, and it moved only a fraction. There still was some good news. I had a strong term for the schools in Britain to look at. I also had a professor for a recommendation. I was on a roll, because my grades in my next term were looking just as good. I had sent in my transcripts and application. I had given all my recommendation forms to Dr. Silver, Dr. Nobler, and the staff at the horse farm to send. The recommendations were confidential. To this day, I still have no idea what they said.

"Good job on those grades last term, mate! I have also looked at your recommendations here, and they are strong, very strong indeed. I do not want to get your hopes up, but you have a slight chance. These are among the strongest recommendations I have seen. Your grades, though, well, those are weak. If you got accepted, it would be a record for the lowest I've seen go through. I have everything, and you should expect to get a letter either way at the end of May. Once last thing: I am going to do you a favor. I will put a good word in for you. Keep your fingers crossed, mate!"

I hung up the phone with Ryan Kelly, and all I kept thinking was "weak grades, lowest I've seen, slight chance, and keep your fingers crossed, mate." It sounded like my application was like a half-court shot at the buzzer. I started thinking, "I'll just apply again next year when I apply to all the US vet schools."

Second term ended, and my grades remained strong. I had signed up for summer term because I had to catch up with my classes. *Calculus the Rematch* and *Calculus the Revenge* had put me behind. Also in order to boost my GPA, I lightened my course load in that first term. Summer was time to pay back that debt. I had statistics, business, a physics lab, and Organic Chemistry II. Dr. Nobler wasn't teaching the summer session, so I had Dr. McMean. It got worse; the class size was easily over a hundred.

Statistics was another winner. The class size there was over two hundred, and the professor was horrible. He mumbled and his lecture pace was extremely fast. *Ballistic* is probably a better word. The last catch for summer was the lectures were longer to make up for the shorter term. You were also covering more material in a shorter time frame. I knew it wasn't a good sign when, despite this, the statistics professor was finishing lectures fifteen minutes early. After the first low-grade tests in Organic II and statistics, the summer term was off to a miserable start. I started to feel like a team that had just struggled to catch up at half time, only to be blown out in the second half. The end of May came and went, and there was no letter.

The low point was in June at physics lab. I was talking to Mike before lab started. Mike was a pre-med student. I was not close friends with him, and we would rarely hang out outside of class. I met him in a class in first year. We seemed to end up in a lot of the same classes, and we would always BS before class started, physics lab being a perfect example of this. I was telling him about my applications to Britain and that my letter was long overdue.

Apparently two pre-med haters sitting in the row in front of me heard the whole conversation. One of the haters then blasted, "Vet schools in Britain! Who the hell applies there? That has to be about the dumbest shit I have ever heard?"

"You hear about that, Greg?" he turned and asked his hater buddy who just shook his head. "Aren't you still like in third year? You have got no chance! None."

"We'll see about that, bro! If I get in, you won't see me at the final exam. 'Cause this lab isn't required in Britain!" I fired back and added a hand gesture with a middle finger to emphasize my response. I remember thinking, with the letter long overdue, that was probably the worst comeback of my life. I would end up paying for that remark and the gesture, and it wasn't going to be pretty.

It was the afternoon of June 13 when the phone in our apartment rang. "It's for you!" Heath yelled out after answering it. Thinking it was one of my friends, I was about to answer, "What's up, bro?" But I chose just a simple, "Hello." (Good choice).

"Hello! How are you doing? I have some good news for you regarding your application!" It was Ryan Kelly. I immediately knew the answer. Without receiving a letter by now and just a phone call it wasn't the news I wanted. I already heard him saying that if you apply again next year, you will have a really good chance of getting in, "mate."

As soon as I finished the thought, he restarted, "You have been accepted at Edinburgh. It was your recommendations that won them over. Congratulations, mate! I'm sorry for the delay. We have been quite busy here. I knew you'd be anxiously waiting, and I wanted to call you personally. You should receive a formal acceptance in the mail next week."

I thanked him profusely. It was like I'd won the lotto. My chances were probably close to the same.

He continued, "You don't have to let me know this moment. I know it can be a big decision—"

"I can tell you right now. I'm going. A hundred percent, I'm going! I'll sign and return the paperwork as soon as I get it," I responded before he could finish. That was it, just like that I was in!

June 23

I arrived at the appointment to complete the process of withdrawing (dropping out) from UF. You'd think you could just sign a paper and hand it in or just stop showing up to class, and they'd get the idea. However, it didn't go down like that. I had to meet with an assigned special advisor, and there was a secretary to act as a witness. She even signed all the paperwork. It took place in a large conference room with a long table and a lot of chairs. I didn't know if usually more people attend like parents, but it seemed like overkill.

"I don't know what you guys are used to, but this is going to be a short meeting," I jokingly stated as I sat down. Apparently, I was the only person who got the joke. I told them I was going to veterinary school in Edinburgh, Scotland. I then showed them the acceptance letter. After that, the conversation lightened up, but not by much. They were pretty stiff. I guess dealing with kids flunking and dropping out is not a fun, regular experience. It was a short meeting. After a few signatures, including the secretary's, it was over.

All the hard work and the struggle had come finally come to an end. Heath was right, I did find a way in. He was as pumped up as me. My father was also pretty excited. For the next several weeks, he enjoyed ending phone calls with, "I heard the Atlantic Bridge is only for medical students." I almost forgot. I never made it to that physics lab final. I also never saw the two pre-med haters again.

Culture Shock

OK, what I experienced in Florida was "culture shock for beginners" compared to Edinburgh. Before we go any further, let me also tell you it was the '90s. This was before the Internet really took off. There was no researching Scotland, Edinburgh, the University of Edinburgh, or the veterinary school on Google, no reviews, forums, blogs, or cute online pictures. All I had was a little book that gave an overview of the vet school and the courses year by year. There were a few pages about "Life in Edinburgh," and that was it. I also had a copy of *Edinburgh: The Complete Travel Guide* that I bought in the Gainesville Barnes & Noble. It was printed in the eighties. Just by looking at the pictures of people in seventies clothes and their giant antique cameras, you could tell it was unreliable intel.

After finally blending in at UF, I had to start all over again, except, bad news, there was no blending or even mixing. It never happened. Beyond the NY accent in Florida, it was American accent now. It was recognizable too. The school, grocery store, gym, bar, everywhere, I was a foreigner, or a "Yank" (their cute nickname for an American). I was called it affectionately and, other times, not so affectionately. To people outside the vet school, I was a tourist. To those in the vet school, I was also a tourist, just one who was visiting for five years.

You read that right—five years. Veterinary school in Britain is five years. In the United States, it is four, like medical school. Quick geography refresher: Great Britain (Britain) is composed of England, Wales, and Scotland. They are separate countries, and don't ever call England "Britain" in front of a Scottish person. Also, don't call it *Eden-Burg*. Its pronounced *Edin-borough*. The Scottish people pronounce it *Edin-burrah*. If you're American, just stick with the *Edin-borough*. No matter how many different ways you try to say *Edin-burrah* correctly, they'll find something wrong with the way you said it. It will only make it worse. Trust me: I know.

The five-year duration is only the tip of the iceberg. My first two years there was one exam at the end of the year for the entire course grade. In the later years, the terms were broken up slightly, but not by much. As far as multiple-choice tests, there were none. The exams were all written, in the form of essay questions.

Take anatomy, for example. At the end of the year, the exam was two parts. One part was a spot test. You'd go to different stations with pins in specific cadaver body parts. You would have to identify the labeled part and write it down. You were responsible for every artery, nerve, tendon, muscle, bone, and organ. Not every animal shares the same anatomy. Part two was the essay. Here's how that went: "Describe the dog's forelimb from the carpus (wrist) down. Include all major arteries, veins, nerves, tendons, ligaments, and bones. Be sure to include diagrams and label them accordingly." There were three or four questions like that. They gave you a lined-paper book to write your answer. Those two parts represented your whole year's grade, pass or fail, on one test.

The grading scale was also different. Fifty to fifty-nine was a passing mark. Sixty to sixty-nine was pass with "credit." In this scale, *credit* doesn't mean credit for the class. It was an honor term. Seventy and above was "pass with distinction" which is the equivalent of passing with high honors. No one, I mean no one, got higher than an eighty back then. So basically eighty, that was a like a hundred. Lastly, there were oral exams that were held after the exam.

If you failed, you were called for an oral exam. If you were close by a few points and could show you really knew the material, you passed. If you were greater than five points away, you'd still have to take the oral exam. Even if you showed you were a genius, you still failed. If the final mark was a fail, you could retake the exam before the term started the next year. Fail that and you had to repeat the whole year, including the tuition, that is, if they decided to take you back. Alternatively, you could be kicked out. No pressure.

There was another group of students that had to take distinction orals. Their questions were much harder, and they had to demonstrate that they really knew the work. If they failed their orals, they passed with credit but did not receive the distinction (high honors). They did separate the lists, but there were no scores until later. There would be three lists: pass, pass/fail oral, or distinction oral. In the olden days, we were told by our professors that there were only two lists: pass and oral. For some arrogant students, they thought they had a distinction oral, and it was really a pass/fail one.

The other popular legend: one professor examined a student in an oral exam and asked only one question. "Look outside the window, what color are the leaves, son?"

"Green, sir," the student replied.

To which the professor replied, "Return when they are brown!"

The moral of that story was the professor was so cruel that there was no second chance oral. He was saying, "See you in the fall before the term starts!" In my time, the orals were moderated by professors from other veterinary schools to eliminate any bias and keep it fair.

The students were the other major difference. Most came from England and Scotland. A few were from Ireland, five from Norway, three from the United States, and one from Canada. The difference wasn't only nationality; it was also age. I was twenty-one. Most of the students from Britain were on average only eighteen years old. In Britain for the ages sixteen to eighteen, they can go to secondary school known as "A levels." If they get high marks and score high on the UKCAT test, they can get accepted to veterinary school at nineteen. There were a few students from the UK who went through university, but the majority were from A levels, compared to the United States, where the youngest was usually twenty-one years old and the average age was twenty-four.

Socially, it was like being back in high school. Despite the cultural differences, it made it even harder to fit in and get along. Beyond that, all the young students were extremely intelligent. Genius is probably a better word. Going through the course work seemed effortless for the majority of them. Nothing highlighted this more

51

than during anatomy labs. The young British students would look through specimens and be done in less than an hour, leaving the foreign students behind while we took comprehensive notes and stayed for close to two hours. The majority played the parts of geniuses quite well. Some weren't as smart as they thought, or pretended to be, and ended up on that pass/fail list.

My first year I had to come back "when the leaves were brown" in two of the three courses—biochemistry and physiology. Yeah, it was a rough first year. In physiology, I was on the pass/fail oral list at the retest! Talk about stress and pressure. Getting kicked out or repeating the year were real possibilities. It would be great when all the students in my class were in second year and then saw me and said, "There goes Miller, the dumb American that had to repeat first year. All those Americans must be stupid." Not to mention the tuition. Do student loans cover repeat years? I didn't want to have to find out the answer to that question.

The oral exam was usually the next day. But for this retest, it was three days later. It was the longest three days of my time in Edinburgh. I showed up for my scheduled oral-exam time. I was exhausted from three days of studying and three sleepless nights of stress. The physiology professor looked at me, confused. "What are you doing here, Mr. Miller?"

"I have a pass/fail oral at 9:45 a.m., sir."

"You do? I don't think that's correct. Oh, I see your name here," he said, looking at his clip board and using his pen to cross it off the list. "That was a mistake. You passed actually, passed by more than seven points, in fact. No oral exam for you today, lad. Good show. You passed!" he replied.

I was too relieved to get upset over the days of agony that mistake had cost me.

My first year taught me how to study, really study. I evolved quickly after that. I learned how to absorb and retain large amounts of information. I would recopy my class notes every night and then test myself with a blank paper to see what I could remember. Nothing shows you how much you don't know than a blank piece of paper staring back at you. I'd use diagrams, short outlines, anything I could to help me retain the information. Toward the exam, I would repeat the process with the whole term worth of notes. I would do bulk sections and make a schedule to cover all the information before the exam. It was a system that I'd use for the next four years. It worked. I never had another resit exam after the first year.

Dogs Don't Have Strokes!

When I was first accepted into Edinburgh I had researched its reputation. As one of the oldest veterinary schools in the world, its reputation was excellent. I had asked Dr. Silver about British vet schools when I was applying. His response was the classic vet joke: "You know which vet school is the best? The one that you get accepted to!" When I told him I got accepted to Edinburgh, after repeating that joke again, he told me that it was considered to be a great vet school. Starting out, I already knew it was a strong school. Despite that, the punchline would be in the back of my mind, "The one that you get accepted to!" thinking, if I slid into it, how excellent was it really?

The answer is, it truly is excellent. After being in practice, I have come to appreciate how great a school it actually is. There are a lot of factors that made it great. The approach to teaching wasn't just having you memorize information. Edinburgh taught me how to think critically. How to break down even the most complicated cases and make them simple. A lot of that came from problem-based learning. In this style of teaching, we would be presented cases to solve in small groups. This didn't just happen in our last year; we were taught like this from the beginning. The other major factor was the professors.

All of them were excellent. Even the worst professors were still good. They were all practical. The majority had been veterinarians and worked in private practice before going into teaching. Everything we were taught was taught from what it would be like in the real world, in other words, what tests and equipment you would have access to in your veterinary practice. In some of the US vet schools, this isn't always the case. Some professors don't have the real-world experience and don't approach things practically. They have spent their careers in the world of academia. Instead, some vet students are taught to run tests and approach cases in ways that wouldn't work in general practice. At Edinburgh, we were taught,

"This is the ideal way, but this is the way you are probably going to have to approach it in your practice."

The best example of this was Dr. Ben Smith. He was tall, thin, with short, brown, curly hair. He was in his late thirties. He was perpetually energetic and never in a bad mood. He always walked around the farm-animal hospital in blue coveralls and rubber boots. Most of the farm-animal hospital was outside, and even in cold weather he was in the short sleeves of his coveralls with just a T-shirt underneath. On rare occasions when it was freezing cold, he'd wear a zip-up fleece jacket. He had the typical farmer's tan, and for all purposes, he looked like one. He was modest and down to earth. By the way he acted, you would never know that he was Dr. B. D. Smith. It was like they were not the same person. Dr. B. D. Smith was an academic genius. He had advanced degrees in numerous specialties in veterinary medicine. He had also written a *ton* of scientific papers and books. Dr. Smith was well known and highly respected in farm-animal medicine. Since he was so modest and straightforward, all the farmers he met loved him. If farm-animal medicine had a rock star, he was it.

What made him truly great was his practicality. The majority of his scientific studies and articles were written about things that could be actually done and used in the real world. His approach was always how to make diagnosing and treating things easier for the vet in the field. He also applied this to teaching students. He constantly preached the expression "less is more." He also used it jokingly, asking students, "Have you read *Cosmopolitan* magazine this month?" He'd then continue, "If you read it, you'd know less is more." Where most professors would be referring to scientific journals to quiz students, he was making a joke referring to a trendy magazine as if it was a medical journal. But underneath this joke, there was a valuable lesson, a golden rule that I still use today.

I have seen other vet schools, hospitals, and veterinarians have a different philosophy, the opposite one, where the more medicine and treatments they can prescribe, the better it will be. This isn't true, and that was Dr. Smith's point. Coming up with more treatments and more medication doesn't make you a better doctor. Using less, and getting excellent results, makes you a better doctor. It was important from a farm-animal standpoint to prescribe what a farmer is going to have time to do and afford. The same applies to a pet owner. A busy mom may forget to give tons of different pills. Maybe she can't afford six different pills for two weeks. Dr. Smith wasn't preaching to cut corners. No, the point was to eliminate what wasn't necessary. Less is more means doing an outstanding job and being practical.

If you hadn't already figured it out, "less is more" was also an underhanded reference to a male's anatomy. Twenty years ago, it wasn't always politically correct. There were no "safe spaces" to hide either. Let's say you were called on and didn't know the answer. If you were lucky, they'd ignore your answer and move on to the next student. If you were unlucky, or your answer was really bad, then you might have a problem, a *real* big problem. That's what happened to Liz Masters after a cardiology lecture in our fourth year.

After the lecture, we broke into smaller groups of twenty students. Our class size back then was just over a hundred students. In the smaller groups, a professor would present a medical case related to the lecture we'd just had. It was an example of problem-based learning at its finest. It was like a think tank where we would work through a case. We'd have a whiteboard, and the professor would jot down notes. The professor would write down the history and signs. We sat in a circle, and he asked questions in the order we were sitting. Sometimes he flipped roles and he'd be the pet's owner. Then we'd ask questions or request tests, and he'd give us the answers or results.

We had Dr. Geoff Walsh. Unlike the other groups that day, we got the professor who had just given the lecture. He was in his early forties, tall, and in great shape because he liked to run. Because of this—and he still had all his hair—he looked a lot younger. He kept his hair short and parted to the side. He was well dressed, except he rarely wore a tie. Instead he wore a long-sleeved shirt, rolled the sleeves up to his forearms, and left the top two buttons open. He was a veterinarian at the hospital portion of the veterinary school. When he wasn't teaching, he was seeing complicated cardiology cases. Cases referred to vet school for a second opinion. He was a specialist in cardiology. Dr. Walsh had written numerous scientific papers, and he was well known in Britain and even the United States. He was from London, and he had a distinct accent. He also liked to joke around. He'd commonly pepper his lectures with slang, as though he was on a London street corner. When the situation required, he could be the complete opposite, and drop the slang as if he had it on a switch. He was always in a good mood and laid back. However, if you messed up, all bets were off.

Liz Masters was one of those younger students from England who got accepted early. She was smart, no doubt about it, but she acted as if she was a genius, and that was a stretch. She was stocky and short, and she wore wire glasses. Her hair was always in a ponytail, from the first year until we graduated. Any subject, material, or concept that you were struggling with, she'd be sure to tell you how simple it was. That usually happened when you were in the middle of talking to someone else about it. As one professor jokingly pointed out one time, "If you keep it up, Miss Masters, you will find friends to be quite a limited resource." I guess if I could have picked someone for *it* to have happened to, she'd have been in my top three. It went down in our fourth year.

"So, Miss Masters, we have a history of a dog with episodes of collapse. Can you give us something for our list of possible differential diagnosis?" Dr. Walsh asked, standing in front of the whiteboard, pointing his red Sharpie pen at her.

"A stroke," she confidently fired back. I instantly knew, as did everyone in the room, that that was the *wrong* answer. It was more than wrong, and she'd have been better off not answering at all. In fact, almost any other answer would have beat that one. Instantly Dr. Walsh's expression changed and not in a good way. All the happiness had been drained from his face and replaced with anger.

"*Stroke?* Did you just say stroke!" he yelled back at her.

By this point the room had gone into pin-drop mode. Anyone who had been daydreaming was now wide awake. For most of us, we could already sense the show was about to start, and we all had front row seats. What we didn't know was this event would be talked about for the days, weeks, and even months yet to come.

"Yes?" she said quietly. It was almost as if she had been hoping it was a test and he had been going to reward her for sticking to the answer.

"You have to be kidding me! *Stroke!* I just stood up in front of you in lecture not thirty minutes ago—*thirty bloody minutes ago*, to be exact—and told you dogs *don't* have strokes! And the first word out of your mouth here is *stroke*? *Rare!* In fact, *never!* That is a disease that *man* gets! Dogs don't get clots from eating bloody fish and chips every day! Arterial sclerosis is a disease of man. Dogs don't have strokes! You do know the difference between a *dog* and a *man*, Miss Masters?" (That line right there would be used against her by students from then on.)

She slowly was nodding her bright red face up and down to answer yes.

"Good. At least you learned that in first year! I am blown away, *gobsmacked*, that your memory is that poor! I can't believe that you're an idiot! It cannot be true. No, you were either daydreaming or talking about what pub you're going to tonight. Anything! But that! You would have not been admitted here and made it all the way to fourth year if you were that bloody thick! Miss Masters, I want you to sit there and pay attention. And for God's sakes, when I reach you again, that answer better be intelligent!"

"Stroke?" he muttered, shaking his head. I thought I heard him then say, "You donkey!" but I could not testify to that. Around the room he went, without any more drama. It was as though it had never happened. Liz Masters just sat there motionless like a statue, with a blank look on her face and holding back tears. From time to time, the students would stare at her, waiting to see if she'd break down, but it never happened. By the time he reached her a second time, she'd recovered, but she still didn't look right. Luckily for her, Dr. Walsh didn't hold grudges, and she had the right answer.

The exams and the constant questioning were a lot of stress. By questioning, I mean being put on the spot in front of a group your classmates with two possible outcomes: one, getting the question right, or, two, looking like a complete idiot, with the possibility of the professor using you as an example. It might not have been as bad as the Liz Masters experience, but nobody likes being wrong. Regardless, whatever you got wrong, your classmates (at least the ones you didn't like) were quick to tell you, "I can't believe you bloody didn't know that one. I wish I was called on for that." By fifth year, I was ready to graduate and move back home. I was talking (complaining) about that very thing to some of my friends when Dr. Reid heard me.

Dr. Dave Reid was from Canada. He didn't have any special degrees or advanced training; he was a horse vet with experience—a lot of experience. He had worked on busy racetracks in Canada and the United States for the last ten years. He grew up in Canada, but his family was from Scotland. A close uncle of his had been diagnosed with cancer. He wanted to move back to Edinburgh to spend time with him. When he flew over, looking for a job, the dean had liked him instantly, and Reid had been hired on the spot. Without advanced degrees, he wasn't always popular among all the faculty. A lot of the vet residents pursuing their advanced degrees were jealous that he was held in such a high regard without any specialty degree. The reason the other faculty liked him was the same reason the dean hired him. He was knowledgeable, practical, and a great teacher. There wasn't anybody nicer or as patient as Dr. Reid.

"I don't understand why I always hear you guys complaining," he said as he interrupted our conversation (last complaint). "You guys have it easy—believe me. All you have to worry about is passing exams and what pub you're going to. Wait till you get out and have to worry about real cases, your job, your boss, and paying bills. Trust me: enjoy it while it lasts! This is probably one of the best times of your life right here."

"Yeah, right, Dr. Reid. That's a good one," I replied as he walked away. "What's he thinking?" I started back with my friends. "I can't wait to get out of this place and back home. Graduated and done! It will be fun being in charge of my own cases, not getting grilled all the time. That's fun. Not this stress! What vet school did he go to? He must have been some kind of genius and cruised through. That's probably why they hired him."

Little did I know, he made some really good points back then. In fact, now I'd have to agree with him, especially if you asked me that ten years later, after the case with the service dog.

The Service Dog

Service dogs are working dogs. They are trained to provide assistance to an individual with a disability. They may help lead a blind person, retrieve objects for a person in a wheelchair, or alert a deaf person to important sounds. Some dogs are taught to alert to the sounds of the telephone, oven timers, alarm clocks, smoke alarms, and even a baby's cry. Service dogs can also be trained to detect when a person with epilepsy is going to have a seizure thirty minutes before they have one. They can also be trained to detect low blood sugar levels in a diabetic.

A therapy dog, on the other hand, is a dog that is used to provide affection and comfort to people in hospitals, nursing homes, schools, hospices, and to people with autism. Their gentle disposition and laidback personalities allow them to qualify for the job. Therapy dogs are usually not service dogs. Theoretically, a dog could serve as both, but this is not common.

Then there is a fad (scam) that is becoming more common, especially with old people (sorry, grandmas out there). They feel that they are entitled to bring their dogs (precious babies) everywhere. In order to break the rules of the No Dogs Allowed signs, and polices in some public places, they run a scam. The scam is they go online and order official-looking dog vests for their precious babies. Then they outfit the precious baby with said vest, and—bingo!—anytime anyone stops Grandma, she points out the vest. She claims some fake, usually "stress"-related, illness, and they leave her alone. This is not cool, Grandma. Not cool! It takes away from real service dogs, and thankfully a lot of states are now cracking down on Grandma's scam. More and more communities are establishing laws punishing faking a service dog with fines, or even jail time. Service dogs are not considered pets. In my opinion, for their owners they go way beyond that definition. That could not have been more true with Willy and Katie.

Willy was a three-year-old golden retriever. He was big, well-muscled, and weighed ninety pounds. Willy looked like a show dog. He could not have been more friendly and laid back. Service dogs are selected, and not all dogs pass. I don't know if they actually hand out scores, but if they did, Willy's had to have been close to perfect. His owners? That was another story. He was owned by a husband and wife who were both attorneys. The Pfeiffers were not what I considered friendly. They were always short with me and in a hurry. They showed *zero* emotion or personality in the exam room. Every time I was in there, it felt as though I was being interrogated. All their questions were appropriate questions most owners would ask, but the way they asked them was as if I was on trial. No matter what I said, their expressionless faces made it seem they weren't satisfied with my answer.

Willy's real owner, as far as I was concerned, was Katie. Her parents might have paid Willy's bills and called the shots, but in my mind, I worked for Katie. Katie was twelve years old and had cerebral palsy. Cerebral palsy is a disorder that affects muscle tone, movement, and the ability to move in a coordinated way. Some cases can be very severe. Katie had good use of her upper body, but she had difficulty walking. Because of this, she was in a wheelchair. Her communication skills were minimally affected, and unlike her parents, she was a socializer. She was always happy to see me and loved to talk. She talked to me about everything, but the main thing was always movies. She was an avid movie fan. If I had seen it, she wanted to know what score I'd give it on a scale of one to ten and what my favorite parts were. If I hadn't seen it, she'd tell me whether I *must* see it, or if it was what she'd call *fair*. If it was really bad, she'd shield her mouth from her parents' views and mouth to me, "It sucked!"

Willy came in on a Tuesday morning at 8:30 a.m. The computer note read, "Drop-off exam. Vomited several times overnight. Depressed. Call Katie in afternoon with an update." A drop-off exam is just that: the owner drops off the pet. We do our exam, test, and what needs to be done. We call them and go over the results on the phone. Then the owners can pick up their pets later or, for most clients, after work.

Mrs. Pfeiffer was sitting in the exam room staring down at her BlackBerry when I walked in. Mrs. Pfeiffer was short and thin, and her blond hair was cut like a boy's and parted to the side. She wore her typical business suit and high heels. She was always very professional and gave the appearance of being strictly business. She was furiously typing on her BlackBerry, and had already started her workday. It was a school day, so Katie wasn't there. Willy was laid out on his side. He barely acknowledged Jen and me as we walked into the room. Willy was extremely laid back, but I could tell instantly he was sick. I got a rushed history from Mrs. Pfeiffer. She acted as though she was doing me a favor answering my questions and I had already wasted her time making her wait to get them. She signed our drop-off consent form and left Jen, Willy, and me in the exam room. It felt as if I was out to dinner with someone and they had left in the middle of it.

The history was simple. He'd vomited five times overnight and had been extremely lethargic. I asked about table food, twice, and she told me, "*None!*" both times. Actually, the second time she reminded me that I'd asked that already. Working on Willy was always a pleasure—he was a model patient, the exact opposite of Cuddles in every way. Willy was the type of dog that I pictured working on in vet school. There was only one catch with Willy, and it was a big one. Willy had a job to do, and someone who *really* needed him. You'd better figure out what was wrong and fix it. Fix it immediately so he could get back home. The clock had started ticking as soon as Mrs. Pfeiffer signed the form.

Willy's blood work came back normal, aside from some mild dehydration. I took X-rays on Willy to look for a foreign body (something he ate but shouldn't have, like a toy), and they were normal. I took X-rays to be thorough, but the likelihood of service dogs chewing up things and swallowing them is small. Despite the attorney's answer, I still sent out a test for the pancreas to the lab.

65

The plan was to put Willy on fluids and get him out this evening. The average dog we would have already planned on keeping one night, but with Willy we were "on the clock."

We had Willy on IV fluids all morning and afternoon. When four o'clock rolled around, I was getting ready to call Katie and let her know what was going on. Essentially Willy was doing well, and he was going to go home. He already was looking a lot brighter, but I knew he still wasn't himself. It was right then that the speaker on the phone in the treatment area came on and I heard, "Katie is on line one for you, Dr. Miller." I was about to pick up the phone, and just then, Jen opened the door from the kennel area to the treatment area and said, "Dr. Miller, Willy just vomited a small amount of bile."

Even under that pressure, the decision to keep Willy overnight was the easy part. It was breaking it to Katie and then calling her mom that was the difficult, rather painful, part. I picked up the phone. "Hey, Katie, Willy is looking a bit better. However, he vomited again. Actually, just now. I suggest we keep him overnight. If he does well overnight and the vomiting stops, he will go home tomorrow afternoon. I promise."

"It's OK, I understand Dr. Miller. I definitely agree with that plan," she answered. It wasn't what she said but the way she said it. She was depressed. She was expecting to hear he'd be back home tonight.

I explained to her we were waiting for the test to come back for his pancreas. I tried to ask again about any table food. "Any chance Willy could have *accidentally* gotten something that's not dog food?"

She interrupted. "I'm not dumb, Dr. Miller! I listened to your 'lectures.' No table food. I get it. He gets nothing."

I could tell her depression was slowly turning to frustration. It was also the first time I heard her starting to talk more like a teenager and less like a young girl. I changed the subject. "By the way, dogs can also get pancreatitis from other things, like eating cat turds out of the litter box."

"That's nasty!" she answered. Yeah, she was right—that is nasty! It's an acquired taste. Apparently, a lot of dogs have acquired that taste. We deal with that fine-dining experience all the time, and it can cause vomiting and diarrhea. "Willy never goes near Felix's litter boxes. Plus, they are all covered. Thanks for ruining my dinner," she joked.

It was good her sense of humor was returning. I then explained to her that we got a fecal sample on Willy this afternoon just to rule out intestinal parasites (worms). I told her his stool was normal, but parasites can also cause vomiting.

"Well, Dr. Miller if you're trying to put me on a diet, you're doing a great job. Who can eat after all that?" After giving me a hard time, she switched back to being serious. She thanked me and told me, "I'll be happy when he's back home. All this medical stuff stresses me out. Talk to you tomorrow." She wasn't the only one feeling the stress.

I told her Jen would call her mom when she checked on him that night. That was part one over, now to part two. I called Mrs. Pfeiffer. That call lasted less than thirty seconds. "Not tonight. Overnight. Fine. Tomorrow. Call us tonight. Bye." I barely got to talk. I felt like a dry cleaner telling her when her blouse would be ready to be picked up.

10:30 p.m.

It was a long evening waiting for Jen's phone call. In general practice, as opposed to the specialists, we get the simple cases, the ones I like: vomiting, fluids, withhold food, bland diet, done. I had a feeling this wasn't going to be one of those cases. There was no Mrs. Sweet that slipped some secret Chinese food on this one. Something else was going on, and I had no idea what it was. Murphy's law, bad luck, or whatever you want to call it was in on this one. This is not the family to have along for that ride either.

The phone rang; it was Jen. It never fails. No matter how many cases, no matter what the update is, the first few seconds after I answer and I wait for the news, it seems like hours. It feels whoever calls me is talking slow on purpose, even though they are not. I feel it's as if they are reading the answer on a TV game show, pausing for dramatic effect. "Well, Dr. Miller, Willy is doing great! You can tell he wants to go home. He's like a new dog, no vomiting and no diarrhea."

"Good news! You can offer him some food and call Mrs. Pfeiffer with the update. Thanks, Jen." My relief was short lived. My mind started working again. It couldn't be this simple. No chance.

Wednesday

In the morning, it started over again. Maybe it's different for other vets. For me, some of the cases are kids, and I'm the worried parent. The worrying never stops until they are solved and finished. In my mind this wasn't finished. I arrived at work, and the process started all over again. Instead of waiting for "the winner is…" in my job, it's "has Willy *vomited*?" I fast walked to his chart to read the tech's notes in the record. Jen spoiled the surprise before I could read it.

"Willy is doing awesome, no vomiting. He's even been barking, and you know, he *like* never does that. I offered him more food and he inhaled it."

The tests were back and both negative (no pancreatitis and no parasites). I examined him briefly, and just as Jen reported, he looked great. I called Mrs. Pfeiffer; she was at work already. Her phone call went the same way as the night before. This time it appeared that half the stuff she was saying was to someone else in her office. I was bothering her. She already knew her "blouse would be ready at five." Thanks.

68

That Wednesday was a blur. All day, in-between appointments, I was waiting to hear, "Willy vomited." By four o'clock, I just had to look at a tech and they would immediately fire back, "No, Dr. Miller, Willy hasn't vomited. Stop asking! We'll tell you!" I didn't know why they were so cranky. I had only asked a few times. OK, so maybe I did know why they were cranky. I'll admit it; it was more than a few.

I don't know how it goes down in most medical practices and hospitals, but I do know how it goes down in my vet practice. On TV and in the movies, you always see the nurses respond, "Yes, Doctor!" and, "Right away, Doctor!" My practice is more like the comedy version. Apparently, most of my staff assumed the role of the stereotypical wise-cracking, back-talking sassy black nurse who has seniority. My staff all have their moments in this role, but the award for leading role goes to Jen. Jen is not African American, but she did have her DNA test done through the mail, and it did return two percent African American, a fact she likes to remind us about on a regular basis.

It was 5:03 p.m. when Willy pushed his way through the exam-room door. Being a service dog, his reactions are more subdued. It was as if he wanted to jump into Katie's wheelchair but knew better. Instead he rested his head on her lap and licked her hand nonstop. The one body part that couldn't conceal his excitement was his tail: he was wagging it as though he was trying to shake it off.

Mrs. Pfeiffer was, as usual, typing on the BlackBerry. When I went over his tests results and the temporary bland diet, Katie was the only active participating audience member. Finally, Mrs. Pfeiffer looked up and asked, "So what was wrong with Willy then?"

"Upset stomach. Maybe he ate something he shouldn't have. I don't have a firm diagnosis, but he responded to the fluids and seems to be doing great. Sometimes that is exactly how these cases play out."

I don't know who I was trying to convince at that point, Mrs. Pfeiffer or myself. It's true we have a lot of cases exactly like that. At this point, there was nothing left to do but see how he did at home and if the vomiting returned.

"I see," she responded. Her tone was as if she was still in the courtroom, not the exam room. I felt as though I was already busted and she had nothing left to prove. She had already proved the witness had no clue. The prosecution rests, Your Honor. "OK. Let's go, Katie. Thank Dr. Miller, Katie."

"I just did, Mom. Thanks *again*, Dr. Miller," Katie responded. She had thanked me. Her mom had been on the BlackBerry and hadn't heard it.

With that, they were gone. It was only then that I started thinking, "Maybe I was just being paranoid. He actually did look really good, didn't he? He'll be fine." I kept thinking all of that. Except I didn't believe it. Maybe the prosecution was right, Your Honor.

Thursday

I came in on Thursday morning and asked if anyone had heard about Willy yet.

"Yes, Dr. Miller. We called. No vomiting overnight. He ate, but only a few bites. He's doing well, though. Back to himself," Jen fired back, annoyed. It was as if I knew her answer and I'd asked anyway.

One thing bothered me. Only a few bites? Why? He should have inhaled that food. I checked the appointments to make sure the appointment schedule didn't know something Jen didn't—making sure that Mrs. Pfeiffer hadn't just called and the front desk just hadn't told us yet. There was no such appointment.

It was ten thirty, I just finished a yearly cat appointment. I glanced at the computer screen for the third time since eight thirty. This time it was there in the drop-off column.

It read, "Vomited a small amount of food and bile. Not as bright as last night. Mr. Pfeiffer to drop off. Call Mrs. Pfeiffer after lunch, and Katie this afternoon with an update." My stomach twisted as my mind started working in overdrive. As I looked up, I heard Jen say, "You were right, Dr. Miller. Something else is definitely going on." I didn't feel as though I was right. I felt as if I was wrong, very wrong.

There was no exam-room discussion. This is a case we had seen already. I had all the info and history I was going to get. I didn't even see Mr. Pfeiffer. He signed the form at the desk, handed Cassey the leash, and left. Willy's exam was completely normal. He wasn't a hundred percent, but he wasn't as depressed as when he'd come on Tuesday. His recheck blood work was also normal. I also repeated his X-rays. They were normal. There was a questionable area in the stomach. He had eaten last night, so the questionable area in the stomach might have been food. Being a service dog, chewing things up was not in his nature (yeah, I said that already), but still could be possible. The rest of the abdomen was normal, no obvious evidence of a foreign object. I just finished looking at his tests when Cassey told me Willy vomited again. It was eleven thirty, and it was going to be a long day.

We put in an IV catheter and started Willy on fluids. There were three options for Willy. The first was to refer Willy to our local specialists for an expert second opinion and treatment. The specialist hospital is where I send the really complicated cases (the ones I don't like). No doubt, Willy was starting to become one of those. They would check his abdomen with an ultrasound. Ultrasound gives a more detailed view at the organs in the abdomen than X-rays can provide. For a vet specialist, that test would give a lot of information about Willy.

The second option was to do a barium study. Barium is like a dye that shows up really bright on X-rays. We would give Willy the barium and then take X-rays at different times and watch the barium pass through his digestive tract. It was a great way to look for a blockage or a foreign body that didn't show up on a regular X-ray. Unlike metal coins or plastic toys, clothing or fabric toys don't show up well. That's where barium comes in. The last option was to take Willy straight to surgery. When we can see the foreign body, or there are obvious X-ray changes, this is a no-brainer. When we can't see it, surgery becomes a tough decision.

The name of the surgery is an "exploratory." It's just like its name sounds—you are looking around the abdomen to find the problem. If the foreign body is on X-ray, then the exploratory is to find it and see if there is any damage associated with it. When you can't see it, then you're looking for a foreign body that may not even be there. A negative exploratory means you didn't find anything. In that case, you take a few biopsies of the digestive tract and call it a day, with the hopes the biopsies will give you some answers. There is an expression in veterinary medicine: "If you haven't had any negative exploratories, then you're aren't doing enough." It means that even with surgery you have to do the test, even if it comes back negative (normal).

Option one was my first choice. After calling Mrs. Pfeiffer, she agreed, but getting Willy to the specialists today wasn't going to happen. Neither she nor her husband could leave work unless I thought it was an *absolute* emergency for Willy. If that was the case, they could make it happen. Willy hadn't reached that point, but we agreed that by tomorrow if we were in the same boat, he'd go in the morning. It was the first time that Mrs. Pfeiffer sounded more like a mom and less like a lawyer. It was the longest conversation we'd had in a while. I could tell she was starting to really worry about Willy. She wasn't the only one.

I had already touched base with the specialist about Willy before calling Mrs. Pfeiffer. I had talked to them about a game plan for Willy if getting him there that day wasn't possible. With the Pfeiffers both being busy lawyers, I knew that scenario was more than likely. The plan was a barium study. Barium is great in theory, but not all dogs take it easily. They usually refuse to take it. They'll spit it out, and it ends up all over the place. When things don't go easily, we know who gets all sassy.

"OK, get Willy. We are going to do a barium study," I told Jen and Cassey.

"What happened to the specialist?" Jen asked, almost as if she expected me to say, Oh yeah, I forgot about that. You're right, forget about the barium.

"Not an option for them today, maybe tomorrow. He's staying here for now. So the next step is barium."

"Ugh, I hate barium! You don't have to worry, Dr. Miller. It's not like *you* do any of the work, or you're going to get any on you," Jen jokingly complained.

What made it so funny (or not funny if you're the tech) was it was true. When it came to a lot of procedures, like X-rays, blood work, or putting a catheter in, it was all them. What they wouldn't admit was they didn't want me helping for most if not all of them. They knew they worked great as a team, and for those procedures, Dr. Miller had been cut from that team a long time ago.

I've been there; I've tried to help. I told you I was a nice guy. The other times, they'd had no choice; we had been short-staffed and I'd been recruited to the team. The results were always the same. It usually went downhill, and I joked, "This is what happens when you send a vet to do a tech's job." It was really a hidden compliment more than it was a joke. No one can do a job like a good tech. Technicians are the unsung heroes of veterinary medicine.

There are a few ways to administer barium. The first way, that usually doesn't work, is we feed it to the dog. We add a tablespoon of cat food because dogs love cat food. Barium is chalky and not enticing to most dogs, even with the cat food. We tried that with Willy and no dice. The second way, we rarely do unless the dog is laid back and very well behaved. We wrap the dog in a big towel and slowly administer the barium orally. There is a reason we rarely do it this way. Barium is a dye for the X-rays. If a dog fights us (picture Cuddles), it will get all over the place, like our hands (OK, the techs' hands) and the dog's fur. If it gets all over the dog, it will show up on X-ray and then the test is ruined. Despite Jen's dramatic complaining, there is no barium all over the place. The third way is when I come in. If this dog was like Cuddles, it would be straight to option three. We sedate the dog and then pass a stomach tube and put the barium directly into the stomach.

With Willy and two patient techs, we went with option two. He did great. It was as if he knew what we needed to do. He drank it down from the syringes like it was fruit punch. At the end of the last syringe he'd had enough of the chalky barium. He spat out the last bit in his mouth and violently shook his head. It instantly splattered Jen's hair, face, and scrub top. Cassey's right sleeve was also hit. OK, maybe Jen wasn't being that dramatic.

"Dr. Miller! Quick grab a towel and hold Willy! Unless you want to kiss this barium study goodbye!" Jen yelled from our X-ray room.

I ran from the treatment area, which was right next door. I grabbed a towel they had laying there, and handed it to them.

"Sure, now you show up! When all the hard work is done," Cassey quipped. I held Willy while they cleaned up and ran to switch scrub tops.

It was a race for time, since the first X-ray is at "zero minutes" (immediately after we administer the barium). They returned instantly wearing backup scrub tops. They both now mismatched with green tops and blue pants. The barium study had begun.

5:10 p.m.

It's long and arduous procedure, involving a lot of time and X-rays. Fourteen X-rays and six hours later, it was five ten. I was on hold with the specialist hospital, waiting to talk to the radiologist. We were still using standard X-ray films and not the digital ones yet. E-mailing the films was not an option. (When this case took place, I couldn't text them either.) Their hospital is close to an hour away, so the radiologist would have to give me advice based on my description. Without actual films for her to read, she was really giving me advice versus a definitive answer and an expert opinion. The barium had passed through the stomach, small intestines, and large intestines. It was now primarily in the colon. Essential normal, except for a questionable area in the small intestines. A small amount of barium was still there, but not enough to definitively prove anything.

As I was on hold, I heard Jen joke to Cassey, "Yeah, it's a questionable area all right. Dr. Miller still has a lot of questions. I also got a question: How late are we stayin' here tonight?" To make things even more questionable, Willy had not vomited all day. He even started barking again, which you already know, he *like* never does that.

"Hey, Dr. Miller. Long day, huh? Tell me what's going on with Willy. What are you seeing on those films?" Dr. Rogers had come to the phone, and as always, she was in a good mood. She had read a ton of films for me over years. As opposed to human medicine, vets read their own films. If we need a second opinion, we'll send them to the radiologist.

"You can say that again. Not a fun case, that's for sure," I replied. I then went on to tell her about the last few days with Willy and the vomiting. I felt like I was telling her my life story with that long history. I described the X-rays in as much detail as possible. I finished with telling her that currently Willy was doing great.

"Well, Dr. Miller, I don't have any easy answers for you. Barium transit time is extremely variable. Since Willy has been sick, his bowel may not be working as efficiently. It may be slower. They have done many studies on this, and there is a lot of variability. Based on what you're telling me, I'd sit tight."

75

"What about the next films? Should I come back and repeat them tonight?" I asked. The techs are going to love that, I thought.

"That's up to you. Since he's doing well, you'd probably be OK to repeat them first thing in the morning. If that area is gone by then, you've got your answer. Especially if he hasn't vomited. The bad news, if it's still there, that's not a definitive answer for surgery. It's not common, but I have seen that kind of variability. Who knows? Maybe the barium cured him."

She finished with a classic vet joke. After a barium study, if a pet improves, the joke is the barium cured them. It might be coincidental, or maybe the barium helps with inflammation in the bowel. After the phone call, it was possible there would still be a questionable area in the morning. Great. The day wasn't over yet either. I still had two more calls to make. Well, it was one call and talk to two people, so it felt like two calls. This time both conversations were rough. Rough actually doesn't begin to describe them, and it had nothing to do with the way I was treated either.

Katie was a mess. She tried to pretend all the information I was going over didn't faze her, but I could hear it in her voice. She was crying and desperately trying to hide it. Despite the fact Willy had been doing well, it was clear the only words she was hearing were "stay overnight,' "specialist," and "surgery." It was all she could focus on and talk about. She told me that she was staying up late tonight for Cassey's update. Mrs. Pfeiffer had remained in mom mode. If I hadn't known already, this conversation alone would have proved what a good mother and strong woman she really was.

"I completely understand, Dr. Miller. I know you are doing your best for Willy, and I appreciate everything. I know you're aware this is not easy for Katie. She is extremely worried about Willy. It has been a rough day for her. For all of us. In addition to going through Willy being sick…" She paused. I already knew some other news was coming, and it wasn't going to be good. "Matt's father had a stroke last night. He's already flown to New York to be with him.

His dad is going to be OK. We'll know more in a few days. You know how that goes. But he is going to be OK."

I was at a loss for words. "I'm sorry to hear about that. I had no idea. I could tell Katie was upset. Tell Mr. Pfeiffer I'm—actually, we *all* are thinking about him. We hope his dad does OK. Try not to worry about Willy. Let me do the worrying for you guys. I'm really good at it. Ask my staff," I tried to joke.

She laughed briefly and continued. "I'll be fine, Dr. Miller. It's Katie. It's like she's been hit twice. You know how tough she is. She is very good at hiding how she feels. You'd be surprised. It's obvious now, though, she's really upset. I'm going to let her stay home from school tomorrow. I'm going to try and work from home. If we need to take him to the specialist or whatever, let me know."

"He seems to be doing better. No more vomiting. I'll know more in the morning after we take the X-rays," I replied. I actually hoped. I also hoped I wouldn't have to deal with the "variability" Dr. Rogers was talking about.

"Dr. Miller, I know it's late and you want to get home. Cassey can call us when she checks on Willy. We'll talk to you in the morning. It's been a long day for all us. Good night." Even though she sounded exhausted, it was almost as though she was trying to comfort me as well. She wasn't kidding about a long day.

10:40 p.m.

My home phone rang, and I had been praying for "the winner is…no vomiting!" It was Cassey. "Hey, Dr. Miller. Don't worry. Willy is still doing great and no vomiting. He had a big dump of barium, though."

"Well, that's good news. You don't have to wait for me. You guys can go ahead and take the X-rays as soon as you get there."

"Like we ever wait for you. You must be losing it. Don't worry. They'll be hanging there before you walk in. Kinda like they *always*

77

are. I'll call the Pfeiffers with an update. Have a good night." In my veterinary career, I've had some sleepless nights where my mind is working in overdrive. I try to solve the puzzle even though it feels as if I don't have all the pieces. That night was one of those.

Friday

I arrived and the films were already up on the X-ray viewer. The questionable and variable barium was still in the small intestine. It moved slightly, and the amount had decreased, but it was still there. There was some left in the colon, but that was normal. I had gotten all the information from the films I was going to get, but I still stood there staring at them. I was looking at them as though if I waited long enough, they'd change. Jen then appeared behind me.

"Dr. Miller, Willy hasn't vomited, but he's looking depressed, definitely not as bright as yesterday."

"Bring him up! I'll look at him," I snapped back. It was as if I didn't believe what she was telling me, that I'd look at him and prove he was fine. I examined Willy, and he was definitely changed. He was depressed. His exam had also changed. When I felt his abdomen, he immediately tensed up, a sure sign he was painful. I told Jen I wanted to recheck his CBC.

"I got it, Dr. Miller. I'll get his blood right now," she answered immediately. She instinctively knew it was time to switch to team mode and refrain from any sassy comments. To their credit, in the face of an emergency, my staff are more like in the movies.

The CBC showed his white cells had dropped below the normal range, another vague sign that could show that an infection was starting. In the early stages of an infection, the body will use up all the available white cells first. Then later the body will respond to the demand and make a lot more. That's when we see high white-cell counts, indicating an infection. I already knew what was next—exploratory. In this case, it was going to be one of those ones where what I was looking for might not even be there. All the signs were adding up. I couldn't see it, and it was a guess. Plus, Willy is a service dog. Yeah, you know; they never chew stuff up. I had one more call to make before the Pfeiffers, who were on pins and needles with *two* family members in the hospital. It was Dr. DeSantis.

Dr. Maria DeSantis was a specialist in internal medicine. Instead of working at a specialist hospital, she had a mobile practice. She traveled to general practices and did second-opinion consults right there. She traveled with all her ultrasound and other equipment in her SUV. I had been using her services at my practice for over ten years. She had gone to Cornell, and done her residency at Animal Medical Center in New York City, two meccas of veterinary medicine. She was brilliant and well respected among other specialists. She was five two and skinny, and she wore thick-rimmed black glasses. Her black hair was usually in a ponytail. She was from Brooklyn, and her comebacks were tougher than she looked. Those who didn't know her would think she was a nerd, but we knew her better than that.

My staff adored her. They loved her sense of humor and straightforward answers about anything, even if it wasn't related to vet medicine. They loved to see how far they could push the envelope on risqué and off-color questions. Being the male in this equation, I only get limited info on what they asked or what answers she gave. I do know almost every time she left our practice, she'd look at me, shake her head, and say, "Those girls are crazy. They really are a trip!"

I would have loved to have had her look at Willy, but based on our location, she usually needed at least forty-eight hours' notice. It's almost impossible to get her in an emergency.

"Hey, Dr. Miller! How are you?" Just hearing her actual voice and not her voice mail, I was relieved.

"Hey, Dr. DeSantis. I have a case for you. Not as an appointment, I need your opinion."

"No problem, whatchu got?" She asked in her thick New York accent. I regurgitated Willy's life story over the last few days, just as I'd done for Dr. Rogers. This time I added his latest exam, CBC, and X-ray.

"Cut him!" she replied, just as I finished. "If that barium is still there, I'd cut that dog. If it was me. Good luck." Just like that, I got what I needed.

The Decision

Even with the input from Dr. DeSantis, the surgery was not an easy decision. It never is. No one looks forward to looking for something that might not even be there.

"What about that expression Dr. Miller, if you don't have any negative exploratories you're not doing enough? What about even if it's negative and you don't find anything, it's a test just like doing lab work?"

Yeah, that's what you might be saying, and you'd be right. That's what all the professors and surgery specialists would say too. The fact is, that's not how the owner looks at it. At least in my mind, I worry they don't. In my mind, to them maybe it's win or lose. If you find something, then you're the hero. If you don't, then maybe Dr. Miller just put my dog through all this surgery for nothing. Sure, they understand the explanation, but do they *really* get it?

Well, after you've talked yourself into to doing one, you have to live through that discussion again with the owner, in this case, both owners. I called the Pfeiffers. Mrs. Pfeiffer answered on the first ring. I went over the X-rays, his depression, his painful belly, and his CBC. Then I said it. "The next step is to do surgery. I know it's out of character for Willy, and you didn't see it…but it's possible he ate something. It would explain everything."

There was a pause before she responded. It was a lot of information to process, and not what she was expecting to hear.

"Surgery? Really? You really think there is something in there? Willy is with us all the time. I'm almost positive we would have seen him. Plus, isn't that out of character for a service dog?" she asked me in a sympathetic motherly tone.

This is where it gets tough. All the points that you've already been thinking are used against you. It's now where the doubts come back,

81

and the "loser" scenario creeps into your mind. You have to stick to your decision; you have chosen your fate. You have to own it.

"I agree, but that's the next step. That is why the surgery is called an exploratory. If…if I don't find anything, then the protocol is to take biopsies of his stomach and bowel. He could have an inflammatory bowel condition or other immune-related illness, all of which would all show up on biopsies." There was a long pause. I almost thought we'd gotten disconnected.

"If that's what *you* think he needs, we trust you, Dr. Miller. Go ahead then. Do the surgery. I'm sorry, but you are going to go over *all* this with Katie. Hold on. I'll get her."

It wasn't what she said but the way she said it. It was if she was too exhausted to argue. As if it was too complicated for her to process and deal with. The burden of the decision was on me. It wasn't the lawyer I was used to dealing with. It was the mom who didn't know what to do. She just wanted this to all be over.

"Surgery, Dr. Miller! For what? I promise Willy hasn't eaten anything. You have to believe me!" Katie had just come to the phone, and it was more of an explosion than the beginning of a conversation. It was as though the surgery was a punishment, not a procedure. I went over all the details again with Katie.

"Katie, I know it's not an easy decision for you guys." Try being me, I thought. "You have to trust me: it's the next step. It's the right thing to do. It's the right call. I agree with everything you said. He's still a dog, and you'd be amazed at the stuff I've pulled out that people never saw them eat—"

"Not Willy, I'm with him always. Surgery is like a *big* deal. I don't want to put him through all that," she interjected.

"Willy is young. He'll be fine with this surgery. The sutures will come out in ten days, and it will be like he never even had it. It's not like with people. Dogs are way more resilient, especially him."

There was a long pause, I could hear that she had started crying. She tried to compose herself, and hide it.

"Dr. Miller…I have to trust you. Please take care of Willy. Don't let anything happen to him. Call me as soon as it's done…Let me know what you find…I'd like to visit him today."

With that the call was over. No pressure, Dr. Miller. No pressure.

10:00 a.m.

All my morning appointments had been moved or rescheduled to allow me to do the surgery. I was standing at the surgery table. It was surgery time: the gown, cap, mask, gloves, sterile drape, monitors, his fluids running, antibiotics on board—you get the idea. In my practice, we didn't cut corners, like on some reality vet TV shows. Don't get me started on those. No, when we did surgery, it was the way I'd been taught at Edinburgh. Period. No exceptions.

Jen was monitoring anesthesia, and Cassey was on stand-by to "scrub in" if I needed an extra set of hands. I was ready to make my incision and start looking for whatever it was that there is no way this service dog could have eaten. After the scalpel blade pierced his subcutaneous tissue and abdominal wall, I was in. An exploratory incision isn't small either. It's the whole length of the abdomen. For the next month, until his hair on his abdomen grew back, it would serve as a reminder of that decision.

I started feeling around his abdomen to pull out his small intestines, and scan his GI tract. It was at this point that my heart, mind, and stomach felt like I was back at Edinburgh. The exam was over and the pass/fail list was up. There was nothing to do now but anxiously wait for the results. What list was I on? Pass or fail?

I got halfway down his small intestines when I felt it. It was a small lump. I pulled out the section of small intestines, laid it off to the side of his abdomen on a surgical towel. There it was—a two-and-half-inch-long lump, and it felt like something soft inside his bowel.

The good news was the bowel was only mildly inflamed. In other words, whatever this was hadn't damaged his bowel yet. If it had, we would have had to cut that section out then sew up two healthy ends like a plumber fixing a rotted section of pipe. No, his bowel was healthy. I felt relieved that this hadn't been one of those negative exploratories that proved I was doing enough.

I carefully made a small incision over the length of the object, and it popped out onto the towel. It was soft, orange, and shaped like a cone. It was covered in green bile and barium. I put it off to the side, out of the surgery field.

Jen said, "What is that? It looks like a small toy. Where'd he get that? Good job, Dr. Miller!" Jen was legitimately proud. There are no fake compliments from the techs. If you get one, you earned it. I could tell she was as relieved as I was. The Pfeiffers weren't the only people along on this ride. We were all anxious to find out what object had put us through this misery. Cassey ran in grabbed it and rinsed it off in the sink outside surgery. Even Liz left the front desk, when she heard the commotion, to find out.

"It's a carrot toy. Looks like a cat toy!" Cassey yelled out.

"A cat toy! You know whose that is, don't you?" Jen quizzed me. My mind was focused on closing this section of bowel and then making sure I explored his entire GI tract, twice. Now was not the time to get sloppy.

I woke up from my own surgical trance, and answered, "No. Whose?" I didn't process it, even though the answer was obvious. "Felix! I betchu that's the damn cat's toy! Nice, Dr. Miller! I can't wait till you call them."

Jen wasn't being vindictive. It was more of a response to the pressure we had all been under. She also wanted to see the reaction and shock to the mysterious object we'd just found.

11:15 a.m.

The surgery was finished, and Willy was waking up. I threw my cap and gown in the laundry bin outside surgery. I washed the powder from the latex gloves off my hands and went to the phone. Mrs. Pfeiffer answered the phone on the second ring. She must have been watching the caller ID because she knew it was me.

"What happened, Dr. Miller? How's Willy—"

"Hi, Dr. Miller, is Willy OK?" Katie interrupted.

"Katie is on the phone with me, by the way," Mrs. Pfeiffer said, stating the obvious.

"Willy is fine. He is awake and out of surgery. He is not completely awake; he's still a little groggy. He's comfortable. We have him on pain medication. His surgery went well, without complication. I found the problem. There was something in there actually. In his small intestine. It was a small toy. It looks like a carrot."

"That's Felix's, *Mom*! How'd he get ahold of that?!"

"Katie! Stop. Let him finish."

"The good news is his bowel looked good. Sometimes objects can press on the inside of the bowel when they get stuck. It can compromise the local blood supply. When that happens the section of bowel can start to die. Then we have to cut it out and join the healthy ends. That didn't happen here. We made a small incision in his bowel, removed the toy, and closed it up. I looked at everything, and it was all normal. I'm glad we all decided to do the surgery. It was the right call."

"Thank you, Dr. Miller! You really are the best!' Katie screamed. "Can I see him this afternoon?" she asked.

"I don't know, Katie. I don't think that's a good idea. He needs his rest. Maybe tomorrow would be better. Right, Dr. Miller?" Mrs.

Pfeiffer answered before I even had a chance. The way she answered it was as if she was trying to give me a secret message. It was that she didn't want Katie to visit that afternoon. Mom may have the authority at home, but not on my patient. If it was a secret message, I acted like I didn't pick up on it.

"Sure, Katie. I think that would be OK. We can set something up this afternoon. We need to talk about the weekend, though. You guys are going to have to take him to the emergency clinic at around five tonight. This way they can watch him closely this weekend—"

"*No way! No chance.* Mom, we aren't going there," Katie interjected.

"Katie! Let me talk," she continued. "Dr. Miller, I think you remember when we took Willy there. The doctor was kind of short with Katie—"

"More like a jerk," Katie corrected her.

"Katie, you can hang up the phone now. Please. You can talk to Dr. Miller later this afternoon. OK?"

"Fine. But we aren't going there." The phone clicked, and then Katie was gone.

"Dr. Miller, it wasn't a good experience. Katie was right. The doctor was young, impatient, and didn't explain things at all. I'd rather Willy stay there with you guys. There is no way Katie will let me take him there. It just is not going to happen."

"We'll talk this afternoon. I get the message. We'll figure something out. Let me put you on hold, and Liz can set you up with a time to visit Willy this afternoon." I put her on hold, called up to Liz and hung up the phone.

The emergency clinic is the local vet hospital that is open and staffed when we are closed. They see all the emergencies after our office hours, weekends, and on holidays. If we have a critical case that needs minute-to-minute care or a case that needs to be watched

86

closely, we'll send it there after we close. The Pfeiffers had taken Willy there when he cut his side on the corner of their glass coffee table. It was a simple laceration, and the emergency clinic did a good job. The emergency clinic sometimes gets a bad rap from our clients.

Clients get upset because of the long waits, higher prices, and sometimes the doctor's personality. They don't fully appreciate the higher operating costs the emergency clinic has, for instance being fully staffed all night. A few of the clients' complaints are legit, but ultimately the emergency clinic does a good job. When Grandpa was a veterinarian, he'd have to slide in and take his own emergencies. Trust me, the quality of medicine back then wasn't even close. It's way better now, thanks to the emergency clinic. My opinion didn't matter now. Willy was going to stay here and continue to be my responsibility. He wasn't exactly out of the woods yet either.

The surgery sounds simple: Open dog. Remove toy. Close dog. Call owner. Hear, "You're the best, Dr. Miller." Done. Go home. And even better, it's Friday night! It's more complicated than that. That little bowel incision is a potential two-inch nightmare. It can fail. If it fails, the barrier separating some nasty, foul-smelling slime, loaded with more bacteria than a gas station restroom, continuously leaks into Willy's abdomen. From there, the bacteria have a party, wreaking havoc throughout his entire abdomen. That party has a name, and it's called peritonitis.

It's a severe infection, difficult to diagnose, and hard to treat. It requires a second, more complicated surgery, the prognosis of which is not as good. If that incision falls apart, the mortality rate has been quoted as high as 75 percent. The good news, for the average surgeon chances of that happening, especially since I didn't have to fix any pipes, was less than 15 percent. Guess when the highest chance of that happening is? The next three days. Thanks, young, impatient, no-explaining vet who pissed off Katie. I'll just roll on in all weekend and worry about that 15 percent. Don't worry. I got it. No problem.

5:05 p.m.

Katie and her mom were in one of the exam rooms visiting Willy. His IV catheter had been capped off to disconnect him from his fluid line, and we took off his e-collar (plastic cone) for the visit. A blanket had been set up on the floor for him to lie down on. When I walked in, it became apparent that Willy had no use for that blanket. He was resting his head in Katie's lap and intermittently licking her hand and face. His tongue seemed to pop out every ten seconds like it was on a timer. Katie was bent over, cuddling him. She was permanently glued to him. It was a picture-perfect moment. I realized again what I had already been thinking. Despite my complaining, if I had to pick one patient and owner to flush my weekend down the toilet for, it would be them.

I gently told them about all the complications that could happen to Willy in the next three days. Like a lot of owners, they nodded their head as though they understood, but they really never processed the information. Mrs. Pfeiffer was as far removed from the courtroom as I have ever seen her. I don't think she asked one question. Katie, on the other hand, barely lifted her head up, and every OK she said was muffled by Willy's head. At this point, they assumed that worst was over and he'd be fine. Any effort to get them to go emergency clinic would have been a waste of time. It was already a foregone conclusion he was staying.

"Oh yeah. I almost forgot that carrot." I left the exam room to grab the cat toy that was now preserved in a Ziploc bag. For our practice, objects like that are like a rare, precious collectible, something we worked long and hard for to find. The day we find *it*, it's the most popular item in our practice. We'll look at it, handle it, talk about it, say things like, "Where is *it*? Don't lose *it*. Leave *it* there!" After the owners see it (the unveiling), the allure goes downhill, and *it* loses its value dramatically. It returns to the mundane object it once was. If the owners don't take it, *it* eventually finds its way to the trash. This was the unveiling.

What we learned was Jen was right. It was, in fact, Felix's toy. It (supposedly) hadn't left Mrs. Pfeiffer's bed for the entire year since she'd bought it. She had no idea how or when Willy could have grabbed it. He never went on Mrs. Pfeiffer's bed. At some point, the carrot left the bed. Willy found it, and we know how the rest went down. The when and how is pure speculation. From a medical standpoint, it was most likely in his stomach and rolled out right before or along with the barium. Looking back at the early films, I couldn't positively ID it in his stomach. If we had waited, it would have gotten stuck at the narrow hairpin turn on the small intestine. His surgery would have been more involved, and he would have had a greater risk for complications.

The Pfeiffers said their goodbyes to Willy. Cassey took him back to his hospital kennel and put him back on his IV. We laid out his treatment plan for the weekend, including the times I'd meet her to check on Willy. Before I left I still had one last important phone call, one that I'd almost forgotten to make.

"Dr. DeSantis, I'm glad I caught you and not your voice mail. I must be lucky. I wanted to update you on that golden retriever with the barium study. It had a cat toy in the small intestine. We did an enterotomy, and he's doing awesome. Thanks for the advice—it was the right call. I really appreciate it. You're so good, you can diagnose this stuff over the phone now," I joked.

"Yeah, right, I don't know about all that. You're welcome. I'm glad it all worked out. I'm sure he'll do great. Remember: you're the one that had the guts to cut him. I'll tell you, not everybody always follows my advice. The smart ones do, though," she joked back. "Have a good weekend, Dr. Miller. Catch you later."

It did turn out to be a good weekend. Katie begged us on every phone call to send Willy home. Willy had a rapid recovery. He started eating Friday night and barking on Saturday morning (you know, "he like never does that."). My last decision on that case was an easy one. I sent him home on Sunday afternoon. He never looked back.

Cat Day

It was Thursday morning, and I'd just started my drive to the office. I usually try to get there early, and usually I'm the first one there. OK, just kidding. I'm not one of *those* practice owners. My commute to the office is forty minutes. I try to arrive about ten minutes before my appointments start. Mostly it's closer to two minutes after they start. For me, it's a disease that can't be cured. I wasn't always this way. I caught it in my late thirties. My staff has tried, but there is no cure. Don't worry. I'll be OK. Sometimes it will go in remission for several days, even a week, but it always comes back. I may not be punctual, but I set an example in another department—attendance! In the ten years of owning my own practice, I have had three sick days. That's a fact, and my staff will verify it. I'm the iron horse in my practice, even if I start the day late out of the gate.

It was one of those days, and I was running late. Not really late, actually on time for me, ETA eight thirty-two. That day was not the day to be on Dr. Miller time. It was seven fifty-five when my cell phone rang. The ringtone was one I'd set to my practice number so I'd instantly know it was work. I change the ringtone once and a while, but at that time, it was a Katy Perry song. I worked with all women, so the ringtone was kind of an inside joke.

By the way, I have a good staff. I mean, really good. I'm not just saying that because they may read this; it's true. Any problem, cranky client, or other mishap, they can handle it. What I'm getting at is, they never call me. I mean, *never*. If they're calling, it's an emergency, and it's not good.

"Dr. Miller, what time do you think you'll be getting here? We have an emergency that's due here any minute." It was Liz. She already knew the answer—eight thirty-two. I had been out of remission; my lateness had rebounded weeks ago. "About eight thirty, what's going on?"

"It's a cat, Vega Johnson. He is having problems breathing, and his gums are pale. It doesn't sound too good."

"Who is Vega Johnson?" The name wasn't familiar. For clients I didn't instantly remember, Liz would start telling a story, and they'd become instantly recognizable. She'll say, "You know, the police officer with all the tats," or, "You know, the lady whose dentures move around when she talks." (I try hard to forget that lady). Liz had a great memory, especially with our clients. This wasn't one of those.

"You wouldn't remember him. I had to look at his record." That already was a bad sign. "He hasn't been in four years. It says you heard a heart murmur on the record."

He was a one-time client. Hey, I get it. I know not everyone goes to the vet every year. People are busy. Mom has got other stuff to worry about. Cats seem to get the short end of the stick when it comes to regular vet care. Some people think, "Hey, it's a cat, looks good to me. This vet thing is overrated. That exam and vaccines, that's just a scam for vets to make money. Flea prevention? Why are you *selling* me that? My uncle Johnny never took cats to the vet. They never had fleas either. His all lived till twenty back on his farm. I'm just doing the rabies vaccine here 'cause the county sent me a letter." In the case of Luke Johnson, that's pretty close to how things went down four years ago. Vega's record read, "Rabies only. Owner declines other vaccines and fecal test." Obviously, the chest X-rays, ECG, and heart ultrasound I'd recommended were "not happenin', Doc," back then.

"I'll set up the oxygen cage, and put him in as soon as he gets here." Liz was already ahead of me. She worked up front as a receptionist most of the time, but she was a vet tech. In our small practice, our staff rotates, and they like the change. At least most of the time they do. On Thursdays, her name badge says tech.

"Call me when he gets there." I hung up. Now my commute had just turned into an emergency.

Before we go any further, I am going to have to straighten something out. I know what you're saying. "See, Dr. Miller, that's why you need to be there at eight o'clock. Even eight fifteen might have saved you here." You might be right about that in theory. The reality is we usually get one or two of those emergencies a year. Then factor in they don't all come in the morning. I could be in on time (in remission) for a year, and the one day I'm late, this would happen. I could come in at eight fifteen, the emergency would be there at eight o'clock.

For the record, I'm not the only vet like this either. Liz, knowing I may not make it in time, tried to get Mr. Johnson to another local practice. They didn't have a vet there either. She was dropping her kids off at school; her ETA was even later than mine. I was doomed from the start, even if I had left early.

It might be my imagination, but it seems there are more people on the road when you're late. That's exactly how it was that day. Whether it was a landscaper's trailer, school bus, or minivan in front of me, they were all going too slow. A dose of road rage hit when a woman in a red minivan was in front of me. I had been staring at the stick-figure-family sticker on the back window for ten minutes. It felt like an hour. It had a figure family, but it was a Star Wars theme—Princess Leia, Darth Vader, mini Luke Skywalker, Han Solo, and Yoda. They were all taunting me. I hate those stickers to begin with, and I couldn't figure out who each character was supposed to represent in this screwed-up family. I was almost tempted to honk the horn just to get her to speed up. Forty-five in a fifty-five is not cool, Mom. Not cool! It was Katy Perry who saved me. The ringtone woke me from my road rage–induced trance.

It was eight fifteen. "Hey, Dr. Miller, Vega is here. He was open-mouth breathing, and his gums were pretty pale. I put him in the oxygen cage. He seemed to improve slightly, but he's not looking good. He started coughing a few days ago. He also hasn't been eating for the last couple of days. Then last night at about six is when he started open-mouth breathing. Mr. Johnson said we were closed, and he didn't want to go to the emergency clinic." That was pretty explanatory. I thought Mr. Johnson didn't want to really go to any vet.

"Leave him in the oxygen cage for now. If he stops open-mouth breathing, and his gum color improves, see if you can grab X-rays and blood work."

"I'll call you back in a few," Liz replied before she hung up. I made my turn, and Mom was gone, but the traffic wasn't. In fact, it was worse. The traffic had come to a standstill. It's usually not a good sign when you see cars start to turn around into the empty lane and go the other way. I didn't have that option. This road was the only way to get to my office. The list of possible things that could have been going on with Vega was massive. The list was already starting to accumulate in my head. However, heart disease was on the top of it.

I might as well tell you now and get the bad news out of the way. Diagnosing a cat like Vega is hard, sometimes impossible, even for the specialists, that is, until they get out the ultrasound machine and look at the heart. Dogs, they're a lot easier. Heart murmur, chest X-rays, ECG, and we are well on our way. With cats, all those tests can be normal, and they still could have a form of cardiac disease. The definitive test for a cat almost always ends up being an ultrasound of the heart or echocardiogram (ECHO).

The traffic started inching forward, because most people gave up and turned the other way. I could just start to see the police cars, and the ambulance up ahead. It was then that I reached into my wallet to pull out my vet license. This book would be a lot cooler if I'd said, "I went in my wallet to get my badge." But I had to work with what I had. My game plan was to tell the police working this accident what I had going on, and use the license to back up my story. I don't see anyone impersonating a vet and using that story, but you never know what people say to get out of a jam.

As I got closer, I saw the cars turning around had been directed to do so by the police officer directing traffic. Now the people turning around were doing it because it was mandatory. Katy Perry started singing again.

"Hey, Dr. Miller. Vega stopped open-mouth breathing, and his gums are now pale pink instead of, like, white. Jen and I managed to get blood work and X-rays. I have the X-rays. The blood work will be done in ten minutes. I spoke to Mr. Johnson and let him know Vega is stable. How far are you?"

Way to go, Liz, I thought. I could tell Liz was anxious for me to get there. Who wouldn't be? She was running out of things that she could do on the cat that should have been to the vet two days ago.

"Good job. I don't know how well they'll come through. But text me pictures of the films. Bad news. There is an accident, and they're having people turn around. I am going to see if they'll let me through. I'll pull over and check the films in a bit. I'm getting close to a cop now. I'll call you back."

I had to hang up on Liz. I rolled up to the cop quicker than I'd anticipated. I rolled the window down. "Good morning, officer. I am a veterinarian, and I have an emergency at my practice. This is the only way to get to my office." I had my license in my left hand, and I was trying to show it to him, but he wouldn't look at it.

"Oh hey, Dr. Miller! How are you? No problem. No problem. We'll get you through," he said, as he started giving some coded hand signals to the other police offers further down.

"Just drive along the grass. Go slow. Oh, by the way, Bernie is overdue his annual. I'll tell my wife to bring him in the next couple of weeks. It was good seeing you. Good luck!"

I nodded my head as I pulled away and waved goodbye. I had no idea who he was or that he was even a client. I was completely caught off guard, and my mind was elsewhere.

Since I live over thirty minutes from my practice, I don't see clients often. This doesn't always save me from a potential awkward interaction. I'll be getting lunch somewhere or buying something at a store near the practice. To them I'm instantly recognizable, but caught off guard I can't remember their pet. I'll respond with a "How's everyone doing?" I used to have a lot of faith in that line that I thought was pure genius. That was until it failed with Mrs. Carter when she replied, "I still live alone and have gotten any other pets since you put Hannah to sleep." I haven't come up with a better solution and still deliver the same line. Except now, I'm always on edge that it's just a matter of time before it fails again.

It wasn't until I consulted the client database Liz, later, that I realized who the police officer was. "You know who that, is Dr. Miller. That's Mr. Davis. He has Bernie the English bulldog. His wife just had a baby. He's the police officer that has all the tats on his arms."

It was eight thirty, and Katy Perry started again. "Hey, Dr. Miller, don't worry. Vega is actually looking better. He's breathing really hard, but his gums are pink. All his blood work is normal. Did you look at his X-rays yet?"

"No, not yet. I just got through, give me a few minutes I'll call you right back." I made another turn, and now there was no traffic. Because of the accident, the road was deserted. It was like a holiday. I pulled into a gas station and pulled up the text images. The X-rays came out quite clear on the iPhone. It was obvious—Vega had fluid in his lungs. It was difficult to make out his heart because of the lung changes. I called the practice.

"Dr. Miller, I was just about to call you again. I hoped you looked at the X-rays. Vega is open-mouth breathing again, even on oxygen." Liz is not one to panic. In fact, this is probably one of the only times I have seen (heard) her stressed out in ten years.

"I saw the films. Chillax, man!" I joked to try and relieve her stress. Well, maybe it was for both of us. "Get the injectable Lasix out. Get the pharmacology book. Grab a calculator."

"Hold on…OK got it!" Unlike the movies, we don't have all the drug doses memorized. My anesthesiology professor at Edinburgh made us promise to never memorize doses. "Trying to be smart will only get you into trouble. Look it up. Like I do!" What he meant was, it will only take one time with one drug that you thought you knew to have an unfortunate miscalculation. It was crucial for anesthesia, but it could have potentially fatal consequences with any drug. Dr. Clarkston was also teaching another good habit. "Double-check everything. Twice!" That's exactly what I did with Liz over the phone.

"Go ahead and give the Lasix IV. Then put him back on the oxygen. I have no traffic. I should be there soon." The Lasix would start getting the fluid out of Vega's lungs and hopefully help his breathing. It's a diuretic. Basically, it makes the kidneys dump fluid out of the body, including the lungs.

8:55 a.m.

I entered the treatment area and ran directly to Vega's oxygen cage. He wasn't open-mouth breathing, but his whole body was moving up and down with his rapid, shallow breathing. His gums were pink and normal. Jen handed me my stethoscope, and I listened to his chest. His lungs sounded rough, and his heart murmur was obvious. I grabbed the X-rays and headed into the exam room.

Mr. Johnson put his cell phone down and stood up as soon as I came in. The staff had already told him about the traffic accident and updated him on Vega's status. Mr. Johnson was tall and in his late forties. He was thin except he had a large belly that hung over his jeans and big belt buckle. He was also wearing cowboy boots, a button-down short-sleeved shirt and a baseball hat pulled down low. I apologized for being late. I went over the X-rays and blood work. I told him that diagnosing a cat with heart disease can be tough. I also told him we could do an ECG next, but ultimately, he was going to have to take Vega to a specialist once we got him stabilized. His response blindsided me. If I would have bet on what he was going to say, I would have lost.

"Doc, you do whatever you need to do for Vega. I have always liked that cat, but to my wife, he's like her son. I knew I should have brought him earlier. Well, my wife has been getting on me for the last couple of days. I know I messed up. I'm real sorry. Last night I was going to take him to the ER, but everyone says that place is so damn expensive. I figured he'd be all right. But at seven o'clock this morning, he was looking real bad, and they were closed."

I couldn't believe it. What he said didn't match his last visit in any way, shape, or form. His story didn't exactly match what he'd told Liz about last night either, but it didn't matter. It was like he'd found a new religion. His religion was now veterinary medicine.

"It's OK. You don't have to apologize. Vega is stable now. I have to give you a heads-up, though, Mr. Johnson. The specialist is pretty expensive. It might be close to a thousand dollars, more if they keep Vega overnight. It is truly the best care for him, and it's worth it. I understand your decision either way. If you need me to come up with a plan B, I can—"

"No, Doc! I get it. I just got off the phone with my wife. Vega is getting whatever he needs. Money is no problem. I'll take him to the specialist. My brother's dog went there last year to have his knee worked on. I know the exact place."

I couldn't believe it. The reality is, sometimes even the best clients in this situation have to start looking at other options. Not everyone has the money to pay for a specialist. They need a less expensive plan B. If plan B doesn't work, or there is no plan B, then owners have to go the final option, which is the option no one wants to talk about. The option to put their family member "to sleep." It's not easy. It's rough. *Real* rough. No matter how long you're a veterinarian, it doesn't get any easier. For me, it has gotten harder. The emotional toll of going through this so many times can wear you down. It's part of the job, and unfortunately, you have to deal with it. I'm not going to sugarcoat it and tell you that you get used to it. You don't. You never get used it.

This time I didn't have to go through that with Mr. Johnson. It was a relief to hear his eagerness to take Vega to the specialist. I was happy for Vega and the Johnsons, especially Mrs. Johnson who I never even met. It's never an easy conversation. Things also never go down as predicted (case in point). I have also seen clients that I'd be convinced would go to the specialist, and then they decide against it.

I called the specialist. We agreed to hold off on doing an ECG. The ECHO would provide a lot more information, not to mention the Johnsons could save money passing on a test that wasn't going to change our plan.

9:30 a.m.

Vega's breathing had improved with the Lasix injection. He wasn't back to normal, not by a long shot. But he had been stable enough for the forty-minute drive to the specialist. Mr. Johnson was well on his way by the time I made it into the exam room for my first appointment. It was scheduled for eight thirty. Jen had already gone in, gotten a history, and weighed the cat. Since it wasn't acting normal, she and Liz pulled blood just in case. They were trying to do anything they could to help catch us up.

Despite being an hour late, Mr. Burns could care less. He had camped out in the exam room with a copy of a newspaper and a book with a title I couldn't make out. Mr. Burns was old school. He had a cell phone, but he used it only for calls. He had been a client of our practice for ten years, and he was one of my favorites. He was in his late sixties, but he looked much younger. He was in decent shape, but you could tell when he was younger he'd carried more

99

muscle on his frame. His forearms and hands were massive. His arms were covered in faded tattoos. He always wore an untucked polo shirt, jeans, and white sneakers. His sneakers never seemed to get dirty. They always looked brand-new. He was completely bald. He always made the exam room smell like strong aftershave, which lingered behind long after he left.

Ed Burns was from New York City. He was a retired police officer, and he'd worked in New York City around the time I was growing up. We always talked about the bad old days in the seventies and eighties when a lot of neighborhoods were pretty rough. He'd worked in one of the roughest, Hunts Point in the Bronx. He was modest, and rarely he'd slip out a story from when he was on the streets. Like all displaced New Yorkers in the South, we also always compared notes about local pizza. We were both on an endless search to find the perfect pie that'd be like home.

"Hey, Dr. Milla? Rough day, huh? How's that cat doin'? He gonna make it or what?" His New York accent couldn't have been any thicker.

"He's going to be all right. Thanks for being so patient. What's going on with Roger?"

"No problem. Roger has a few issues lately. He acts like he's starvin'. He has been drinkin' and urinatin' a ton. It seems like da guy lives in dat litter box. He's not himself." Roger was his seven-year-old orange cat. It was a tie who loved Roger more, Mr. or Mrs. Burns. Mrs. Burns had passed away four years earlier from lung cancer. Roger was now all he had left. He had always been slightly overweight, but under Mr. Burns's care Roger had gained a few extra pounds. For a cat, that was quite a bit. Despite us trying to get him to measure out his cat's food, like a lot of owners, he went with the keeping-the-bowl-full method.

"Any vomiting or diarrhea?" I asked as I finished examining him.

"No. None of dat," he replied.

"I'm going to grab a urine sample, and Liz already got his blood sample. Sit tight. I should have the results in ten minutes."

"No problem, Doc." He opened up his paper and sat back down.

Some people are shocked when they find out how we get urine samples in cats. We poke the bladder directly with a needle and syringe. Believe it or not, it's quick and relatively painless. Most cats object more about being held still on their side, than getting poked by a needle. For a lot of cats, staying still even longer for a blood sample is worse. We didn't have to worry about that with Roger: he was the perfect patient.

9:50 a.m.

I had a nine o'clock dog annual. It was a two-year old Chihuahua named Ray. It was pretty uneventful, which helped get us back on track. I'd just finished the suture removal at nine thirty on a cat spay when I stepped out and Jen handed me Roger's blood work. More like, she thrust it in my stomach like a football player making a handoff. I grabbed it, and I can't say I was surprised. Roger was a diabetic. His blood glucose (sugar) was 585. Normal is roughly less than 200. Jen stormed off to check his urine. I could tell she was upset, and I knew why. Diabetics have a really good prognosis. But they require a lot of work. There are worse illnesses we could have diagnosed, but Jen immediately felt bad for both Roger and Mr. Burns. He was one of everybody's favorite clients. What I didn't know was how the diagnosis was about to go over with Mr. Burns.

I went back into the exam room. I went over the blood work and the urine sample (normal except for the glucose in it). I showed him the blood sugar and told him Roger was a diabetic. I told him the prognosis was usually very good. It was even possible for Roger to go into remission. Cats can go into remission with diabetes. When I started talking to him about twice-a-day insulin injections, the train went off the track.

101

"Whoa, whoa, Doc. I gotta give him a shot! Twice a day? No chance. That ain't goin' to work for us. How 'bout a pill like they do in people? I can handle a pill."

"There is no pill for diabetes in cats or dogs. It has to be an injection. It's a small needle. It goes under the skin. It's easy. We are going to teach you how to do it. I have even taught little old ladies to give this shot. They have all left here lookin' like pros." I tried to reassure him.

"Doc, I'm just not good, giving Roger a shot. I don't know what it is, but I'm not going to do it. There has got to be another way. Carol, she would have been good doin' dat stuff. She was a nurse. She could handle this."

I was beyond confused. This guy was a hardened NYPD cop who'd worked in the Bronx. He had seen it all, heard it all, and he couldn't poke a cat with a small needle? I was expecting him to bust out and say, "Just kidding, Doc! I gotcha." But that never happened.

Just then Jen busted through the door with the insulin, and the diabetes take-home kit. The kit had insulin syringes, a biohazard plastic box for used syringes, and a handout about diabetes. As soon as Mr. Burns looked all the items in Jen's hands, he turned away and looked at the wall. It was like she was holding a foul-smelling fecal sample. He was visibly upset. We had delivered news he wanted no part of. My mind was scrambling, trying to come up with the game-winning speech. Just then Jen broke in and started talking before I could even start.

"Hey, Mr. Burns. I got some goodies here for you. If I could handpick a patient for all this, it would be Roger. I love Roger! He is so easy to work with. I wish all my cats at home were as good. Believe me. You should see some of the patients we have a roll in here."

I was stuck. There was no way to warn her about what she was walking into. She hadn't heard what he had just said. She bent down, picked up Roger, and placed him on the exam table. She started petting him.

I decided (was forced) to ignore what had happened before she'd come in, and go along with her as if nothing had happened. I was desperate, and that plan seemed as good as any other. I grabbed the insulin needle and drew up some sterile saline. We use saline as blanks to teach owners how to give injections.

Roger walked over to me. Inquisitive as to what I was working on, he started sniffing around my hands. Jen without missing a beat, went over the handout, insulin dosing, and giving injections. I stood there, petting Roger like an audience member, anxious to see if this was going to work. My eyes were glued on Mr. Burns's expressions. His face went through a large variety of expressions, most of which I found impossible to read. I felt like I was watching a roulette wheel waiting for it to land on my number.

Toward the end of her speech, she delivered (stole) my line: "We've even taught little old ladies to do this."

His face was completely relaxed. I knew we had a winner when he volunteered to give the saline without me doing it first. He even gave the first insulin injection. I couldn't figure out how transformation occurred. I did know that when I told Jen what he'd said initially, she'd be taking all the credit for it. I had heard it all before, and I'd be hearing it again, "What would you do without us, Dr. Miller? This place would fall apart. You'd never be able to replace us. You think these local clowns could do all this. No chance!" It was her way to compliment the staff and (let us not forget) herself. She delivered it regularly in one form or another.

It was true we had been less than successful in recruiting new talent. Despite our extensive resume selection and intensive interview process, our results with new hires were always the same. They fell by the wayside for "lack of performance." The best employee we'd hired recently, Beth, had left us to become a paramedic. That was the exception to what we usually ended up with. A classic example was when a client begged us to hire her eighteen-year old-daughter, Christine. After a year of this pressure, and being short-staffed, even Jen gave in. We were rewarded when Christine quit two weeks later in the middle of the day with a note taped to a kennel: "This job is too hard, unfair, and I quit. Thank you, Christine."

She'd left through the back, and we'd never heard from her again. Her mom was still a client, though we haven't seen Christine since.

Mr. Burns scheduled his recheck appointment and left. I told Jen about his sudden change. What he had said right before she came in. I was looking for some scientific psychological explanation, but I never got it. Instead without missing a beat, she instantly took the credit. She started explaining her deep connection with clients and finished with the majority of the lines at the end of that last paragraph. Liz had just come back to the treatment area and heard Jen talking to me (rubbing it in about Mr. Burns).

"I know it's crazy! That Mr. Burns is a diabetic, right?" Liz interjected.

"What? Wait, he's a diabetic! Like he actually gives himself insulin?" I asked.

"Yes! I thought you knew that. Isn't that what you were guys are talking about? That he couldn't give the cat insulin, but could give it to himself," she answered.

"No, we had no idea. We thought he had a needle-phobia, or a phobia about giving his cat a shot. I actually don't know what the hell we thought," I said still confused.

"I know what *I* thought. I thought I gave a great speech, and Mr. Burns loves me. If it wasn't for us, Dr. Miller, you'd be screwed. Face it," Jen answered as she grabbed the next appointment's record and went in the exam room to do her check in.

I probably agreed with most—well, at least some—of that, but I wasn't going to tell her. Ever.

3:30 p.m.

It was another storybook appointment. Not like a fairy tale. Rather, what was written on the appointment told the whole story: Eddie Hasselback, swollen rear leg. Mrs. Hasselback has been treating at home for several days and not getting any better. Would like to discuss treatment options." To the average person that looks like a reasonable appointment, but it's far from that.

Mrs. Hasselback is one of those holistic, or alternative therapy, people. I'm not going to debate the merits of holistic vet medicine here. Personally, I'm not a big fan of that either. But I'm talking about clients who research their *own* treatments and therapies, usually on the Internet. Then they discuss the finer points of these therapies with me, as if they actually have a medical degree. When I say discuss, it's more like a lecture, and they are getting me up to speed on things, treatments, and remedies that I should have learned a long time ago. Obviously, I am behind the modern holistic times, and they are going to rescue my practice. Then, once I implement these natural advancements and modern holistic miracles, it will be life changing.

I walked into the room to find Mrs. Hasselback sitting on the floor. She was holding her black tabby, Eddie, in her lap. I didn't know if our bench isn't all natural enough for her, or she feels the tile floor brings her closer to nature. She was wearing a long, thin skirt with a flowered pattern on it. She had a light-blue T-shirt that was obscured by all the wooden bead necklaces she was wearing. She also was wearing flip-flops. Her hair was long and brown, and she had blue eyes. My guess, she was in her midforties. Jen bent down as she greeted her and Eddie and then lifted him on to the exam table.

"Dr. Miller, Eddie's right back leg is swollen. It's been swollen since Sunday. I have been putting coconut oil on it twice a day. When I say put it on, I mean in the form of a ten-minute massage. I think it's improved because I can see the pus coming out of the hole there. I wanted you to look at it so we can maybe discuss something else to add in to help it along. Before I forget, he's still on the brewer's yeast for fleas."

I had just made it to his leg when she finished talking. His right foot was swollen about three times its normal size. There was a small wound on his foot about an inch in size, and I could see the pus she was talking about. As I was taking his temperature, I saw a flea crawl across his back. So much for that brewer's yeast. His temperature was elevated at 103.5 (normal in cats and dogs is 101.5, give or take a degree). This is a very common injury in cats. They get bit by another animal or puncture their skin somehow. The area gets infected, swollen, and then becomes filled with pus. Also known as an abscess, the treatment is simple, and the prognosis is excellent—that is, for people who actually believe in modern veterinary medicine.

"It looks like Eddie has an abscess here. The hole here is either from the initial injury, or sometimes when the pus builds up, it will rupture on its own and start to drain. I recommend we start Eddie on antibiotics and give him an anti-inflammatory injection for pain."

Normally, I don't have to recommend anything. For most people, it's a foregone conclusion, or rather, common sense. Bacterial infection equals "I need antibiotics." Simple. With Mrs. Hasselback, it was a discussion. Luckily Eddie was up to date on his rabies vaccination. I gave up talking to her about other cat vaccines years ago. I figured if the pediatrician couldn't get her to vaccinate her son, I had no chance on the cat. Right before she started her discussion, Jen put Eddie back on the floor and slipped out of the room. She wanted no part of suffering through this. It was right about then I was wishing I could go with her.

"Dr. Miller, I don't know if I'm a big fan of antibiotics for Eddie. It looks like it's already improving. I don't want to upset his natural bacterial balance by giving him those. I was thinking of adding in Epsom salt soaks to help drain the pus. I also was going to increase his brewer's yeast to help kill the bacteria. What do you think?" The discussion had begun.

"Mrs. Hasselback, I understand your concerns but if we want to get rid of Eddie's infection, we are going to need antibiotics. It's really straightforward. If we don't, it's going to get worse. I would get him started on antibiotics immediately. None of those things you mentioned are going to address his pain." I thought that was a pretty clear, solid argument. But apparently it wasn't.

"It has been improving. I have to disagree with you, Doctor. I think my massages comfort Eddie quite a bit. His limping doesn't seem as bad when I'm finished. It's funny. When he is due a treatment, he comes up to me like he knows it helps him. I am disappointed that you don't have anything holistic to offer. Those treatments are kind of...old-fashioned."

"I don't know why you get the impression they're old-fashioned. Antibiotics are the mainstay of modern medicine. If ever a case needed antibiotics, it's this one. I'm sorry, Mrs. Hasselback, but that's my advice for Eddie. I can't force you to do it, but that's the only treatment I would recommend as his veterinarian. I am going to have Jen get you a treatment plan."

With that I made my exit. I'd had my fill of her holistic debate. I figured I'd leave before things started getting heated.

The "treatment plan" was our version of an estimate. It was a way to break down what we recommended and how much it would cost. For complicated treatments or expensive surgeries, it helped owners make decisions. For Mrs. Hasselback, I was using it to force her to make one. It was my chance to get a medical grip on this situation. She could accept my treatment plan, or she was on her own. Jen printed out the treatment plan, which consisted of antibiotics, a pain injection, and a small e-collar to prevent him from licking the affected area. Jen went in the room and quickly returned two minutes later. "She'll do it."

Before you think Jen has got some kind of great client skills, trust me: it wasn't that. At least not in those two minutes. Mrs. Hasselback folded to modern medicine. Deep down, she knew her holistic remedies weren't working, and she was desperate. I don't know how many victories her pediatrician has racked up, but this was a win in the vet column. In this case the real winner was Eddie.

Follow-Up

Eddie did great. At his recheck two weeks later, Mrs. Hasselback told me that she'd started him on apple cider vinegar. She informed me that after they'd left, she'd noticed Eddie had a few fleas. She said they must have come from our exam room. Normally, brewer's yeast would kill fleas, but all the chemicals (flea prevention) we use in our practice had made these particular fleas resistant to brewer's yeast. She told me that if my clients wanted the dose for apple cider vinegar, it was online.

Roger did great, and we got his diabetes regulated. Jen still takes credit for pretty much everything with Mr. Burns, including his most recent decision. He adopted a white Persian cat he named Wendy. Mr. Burns and I still have not found the perfect New York pizza.

Mr. Davis did bring Bernie in for his annual, two months later. I didn't forget his name when I saw his appointment on the schedule that time. When Liz told me, "He's the cop with the tats that got you around the accident last month!" I remembered him instantly.

Vega's news was not as good. Like all cats with congestive heart failure, the specialists told the Johnson's his prognosis was six months. The Johnsons never gave up on their new religion— veterinary medicine. They gave every pill, followed every direction, and went to every recheck. Vega made it eight months when he passed away. A few months later they got a chocolate Lab puppy they named Moose.

After that emergency, I thought about coming to work earlier. I turned over a new leaf. Even my staff was encouraged that the emergency would shock my late disease into remission. Surely if anything could scare me straight, it'd have been that day. That time, I rebounded for three weeks. I still arrive at exactly eight thirty-two.

The Second Opinion

A true second opinion is received at the specialist. It's an expert opinion, usually on a complicated case. There are specialists in many different areas of veterinary medicine. As veterinary medicine has become more advanced, there are a lot more specialists and specialties than when Grandpa was a vet. We have specialists in internal medicine, surgery, ophthalmology, dermatology, radiology, neurology, oncology, behavior, and even dentistry, just to name a few. After vet school these vets do (on average) another three years of training in their chosen fields. They have to take exams and go through a process to get certified (boarded). At Edinburgh, we were told, "The general practitioner is a mile wide and inch deep. Where the specialist is an inch wide and mile deep." In other words, we know a little about everything. The specialist knows a tremendous amount about their specialty.

Our second opinions are somewhat different in general practice. We are asked to give opinions on other vets that are equal to us in qualification and knowledge. In my practice, they fall into two types of appointments. The first is when the other vet is on the right track and the client wanted to double-check what they were told. The second type is where the vet is on the wrong track. The client has finally realized that not all vets are created equal, and maybe it might be a good idea to find another vet. We don't get second opinions often, but when we do, they usually are the second type. In rare circumstances, we'll get a great long-term client this way. Usually, we get those other people who fall into the not-so-great category. Usually the previous vet has jaded them, so I then receive their misplaced backlash of mistrust. Immediately, I face intense scrutiny, and it's up to me to win back their trust in the veterinary profession.

I don't like second-opinion appointments. I'm not a big fan of checking someone else's homework. Trying to explain why the other vet is approaching things the wrong way makes them even more painful. No offense, but if they didn't figure out something was wrong after going to this other vet for months or years without any results, then they need more help than I can offer. Nothing proves my point more than this case.

Mrs. Jackson's second-opinion appointment was for her two-and-half-year-old pug, Scarlet. She had been going to this other vet since Scarlet was a puppy. This vet had been treating Scarlet for the same urinary tract infection for two years. You didn't read that wrong—this vet had been treating this dog for *two years* with little improvement. I guess it took two years of Scarlet having accidents in the house and straining to urinate before Mrs. Jackson realized, "Maybe, just maybe my vet is missing something."

After looking over Scarlet's records, I went into the room with Cassey. This appointment was what we affectionately call a "self-check in." That means I go in and do the check in (get the history). We employ that when we are in a hurry, the history is complicated, or it's Mrs. Sweet. I had a feeling this one was going to be the long, drawn-out version.

Mrs. Jackson was standing in the room, holding Scarlet on a leash. As soon as we entered the room, she extended her hand to formally introduce herself. "Hello! I am Mrs. Cynthia Jackson, and you are?" she asked in her (slightly exaggerated) Southern accent. It was as if I was rude for not introducing myself in the two seconds I had been in her presence.

"I'm Dr. Miller, and this is Cassey." The first thing I noticed was both her hands and wrists seemed to be covered with as much gold jewelry as humanly possible. When Cassey and I shook her hand, the clanking of her bracelets was so loud Scarlet barked in response. Mrs. Jackson was in her early sixties. She had short auburn hair and wore a red business suit with a skirt. On it she had a gold name tag with her name, and the name of some real estate agency.

"I have reviewed your records. Tell me what's going on with Scarlet?" With that one question, I got it all. It was a landslide of information, more than I really needed to know. I'd barely got my questions finished before she started back again with her answers.

After going through Scarlet's medical history and life story, we got an added bonus. She said, "It is my obligation to let you know about me, if you are going to be my baby's doctor." I didn't feel as if it was the privilege that she'd made it out to be. When she started talking about growing up in rural Georgia, I'd had enough. I focused the attention back to the case.

"Looking at the urine tests, Scarlet had crystals in her urine. Those can be a precursor to bladder stones. Did they ever take X-rays of her bladder?"

"Oh, my! You think she has those? If she had them, wouldn't they had told me about it?" she replied.

"He would have needed to take X-rays to find out. Did he take X-rays?" I asked again, trying to get an answer.

"No, I don't remember that. They put her on a special diet for the crystals. Wouldn't that have that helped?"

"A special diet helps dissolve crystals and prevent new ones from forming. It doesn't really work well on larger stones. For that she would need surgery."

"Surgery? Oh, my doctor! Surgery for a lil' infection? I'm confused. I thought you could just give her some different type of pills. I came here for a second opinion on the medication."

"I think it's more complicated than that. That's why all those different pills he gave you haven't worked in the last two years. We have to find out if something else may be causing the infection. I recommend we do blood work, a urine test, and X-rays."

She sat down, and let out a dramatic sigh. "Ok, Doctor. If you think it's necessary, go ahead. Do it. Do it all," she said as she turned away looking at the wall. It was like we were forcing these tests on her against her will. The reality is these tests were needed and were long overdue. A lot of things could have been causing Scarlet's signs. Whatever it was, her previous vet never found it. Spoiler alert: this case wasn't really that complicated. It didn't even need a specialist. Even *I* could handle this one. Handling Mrs. Jackson, that was another story entirely.

Cassey and I took Scarlet to the treatment area. I got a quick exam done. I had opted out of doing it in the exam room. I already realized the best way to take Mrs. Jackson was in small doses. Scarlet's exam was completely normal. She was an awesome patient. Like most pugs, she was extremely outgoing and friendly. Cassey grabbed Jen and they knocked out the blood work, urine sample, and X-rays. I could hear bits and pieces of Cassey giving Jen the run down in radiology. As I was writing up Scarlet's record, I heard Jen laugh and say, "It sounds like Dr. Miller got another *real* winner."

The blood work was completely normal. The urine had a few crystals, but no obvious signs of an infection. Sometimes infections are hard to catch, and she had just been on antibiotics. The X-rays told the whole story. Scarlet had three large stones in her bladder. They were obvious like three small white marbles in the back of her abdomen.

I grabbed the test results and went back into the room. I explained the blood work and the urine. Then I went to the grand finale, the X-rays. I put them up on the viewer and pointed the three stones out to Mrs. Jackson. I told her the stones had been the source of Scarlet's urination problems. I explained to her that the treatment was to surgically remove the stones. The surgery was a straightforward procedure, and the prognosis was excellent.

"Oh, my! How long do you think those have been in there like that?" She was sitting on the edge of the bench with her elbows on her knees and her head resting in her hands. Scarlet, who was lying on the floor beside her, was looking at me like she was following every word I said.

"It's possible that they formed a month ago. But based on their size and her history, I think they have been there for at least a few months. There is no way to tell."

"How did she get them? Was it all those antibiotic pills that caused them?"

"No. It's complicated. It wasn't caused by the pills. There could have been many different causes. It could be genetics, a chronic bladder infection, or even a liver problem. I actually want to do one more blood test before surgery to check her liver."

"I don't know about doing surgery. It seems like a lot to put her through. Isn't there another way to get rid of them? Like another diet?"

"Sometimes a special diet will dissolve smaller stones, but these are too large for that. I think surgery is the best option. I understand your concerns, but it's a common surgery."

"I am going to need some time to think about this. Thank you for your time. That was real...real informative." She stood up and stretched her hand out for me to shake it. She shook my hand again, but this time it lacked the enthusiasm it had the first time. I said goodbye as she quickly left the exam room. It was as if I offended her with my diagnosis. Her exit caught me off guard. I expected more discussion. I left the room and finished writing up Scarlet's record. Like a lot of second opinions, I thought I might have seen the last of Mrs. Jackson.

Second Opinion, Day Three

In the middle of appointments, Liz buzzed back to the treatment area. "Dr. Miller, Mrs. Jackson is on line one. She has questions about Scarlet. I'll bring back the record." I didn't need the record. I remembered all of it. The only thing I needed it for was to document the call. I hadn't expected to hear back from her again.

"Dr. Miller, I have been reading a lot—online. There are a lot of mixed opinions. Most of them seem to agree with you, however." The disappointment in her voice was obvious. "I'm still confused about the whole thing. I thought all the pills and the diet would have fixed this. Are you sure surgery is the way to go for my baby?"

"Without a doubt. If you want a second opinion on what I've told you, then my advice would be to get one from a specialist. I can give you the number. You can take your blood work and X-rays to them. I would not recommend getting another opinion from another local vet. With what you have been through, you want a definitive *expert* answer. I'm pretty sure they are going to agree with me. This is a straightforward case. But, I would encourage you to go. Especially if you're unsure."

"What happens in the surgery?" she asked.

"We make a small incision in her abdomen, like a spay. I then make one in the bladder, remove the stones. We'll keep her overnight on fluids. She'll go home the next day on antibiotics and pain medication. The stones are sent off to be analyzed. Based on the type of stones, we can discuss ways to prevent them from reoccurring. I would also do a urine culture. This is where we send the urine off to the lab to see if there are bacteria there that didn't show up on the urine test. *If* she has one, the lab can also determine the exact antibiotics that work for her infection—"

"Infection? You said you didn't see an infection. Now you know why I'm so confused!" She interrupted.

"Sometimes infections don't show up on a urine sample. Sometimes we need a culture to definitely give us a yes or no answer. With her history of chronic infections and all the antibiotics, I would do a culture."

"She isn't on any antibiotics now. She has been off two weeks. I'm sorry, honey, but you'll have to be consistent in your explanations." She answered back, determined to correct me.

114

"I realize that. But because of how long this has been going on, we need to definitively know if she has an infection or not. It is the only test that will show that. Actually, a culture is considered a standard test for a cystotomy."

"I'd prefer if you just call it bladder surgery. The only reason *I* know what you're talking about is because I read about it online. I don't remember them saying the culture was standard. I guess I may have some more reading to do. I have to be honest, Doctor: it's all so confusing."

None of my explanations seemed to win her over. You'd think she would be impressed. I took those X-rays and found the stones on the very first appointment, all that patience and knowledge. Even most of the Internet agreed with me. I must be on the right track. Not according to Mrs. Jackson. She said she needed to talk to her friends about it and get back to me. I guess her friends trump the specialist on an expert second opinion.

When I hung up, Jen looked up from her cat nail trim, and said, "Man! Why didn't she ask all these questions to her last vet? Her last vet puts her through all that, and you're the one raked over the coals. If I were you, Dr. Miller, I would send her somewhere else. You have been through enough already."

I didn't realize it until later, but that actually was excellent advice.

Second Opinion, Day Five

When I arrived on Friday, I scanned the computer, and there it was: "Scarlet Jackson, bile acids test."

I'll explain it to you exactly as I explained it to Mrs. Jackson. When a dog is in the fetal stage inside mom, its liver doesn't filter its blood. Its blood has another pathway around the liver. This allows mom's liver to do the work of filtering out toxins, storing sugar, and producing protein for her unborn puppy. This special pathway closes down when it's born as the puppy's liver begins to work. In some puppies, this pathway doesn't close down; it's referred to as a shunt. Shunts can lead to bladder stones. It would also be nice to know that Scarlet's liver was OK before we put her under anesthesia.

It took me three times to explain that to Mrs. Jackson. I guess it worked. I can't take all the credit, most of the Internet and her friends might have helped. A bile acids test is simple. The dog comes in fasted. We take a blood sample. Feed it a small meal. Take another blood sample two hours later, and the test is finished. The bile acids test evaluates liver function. If the values are normal, then there is no shunt.

Second Opinion, Day Nine

Scarlet's bile acids test came back normal, which meant a shunt wasn't responsible for her bladder stones. Along with her normal blood work, she'd be cleared to go under anesthesia. I called Mrs. Jackson.

"Mrs. Jackson, Scarlet's bile acids tests came back normal. It's negative for a shunt—I mean, she doesn't have a shunt; her test is normal." I tried to avoid the discussion that came next, but I knew instantly after I said it, it was too late. The cat was out of the bag.

"Dear lord, Doctor, do you confuse all your clients this way or just me? Is her test normal or negative? Which is it?" she asked; the frustration in her voice was obvious.

"I'm sorry if I confused you. Negative and positive are terms we use for test results. Negative means that she doesn't have a shunt. Normal and negative mean the same thing in this case. Her liver is normal. She doesn't have a shunt. This also means she's OK for anesthesia."

"I don't understand why you told me *negative*. If it's normal, you should say it's *normal*. Honey, if I may, I'd like to offer you some feedback. I have been in the real estate business for many years. I am a people person. I know people quite well and how to deal with them. I couldn't sell houses if I didn't. You seem like a fine doctor. But if you are going to be successful, you have to be clearer in the way you explain things. I have a hard time following your explanations. I'm sure I'm not the only one, sugar. A lot of your clients probably feel the same way. They just don't say anything."

Well, the last part may be true, but I'm not taking the fall for it.

"Thanks for the feedback" was my professional answer. The New Yorker in me had an entirely different response. I quickly changed the subject. "Did you decide on surgery? I can have Liz schedule it for you."

"No, that's OK. Can you please tell the girls in the office that I'll be stopping by later today and would like copies of her blood work, including this bile blood test you just did."

"No problem, I'll let them know. If you want to have a second opinion at the specialist, we can give you their information. This isn't a specialist surgery, but you can have that done at their hospital as well. A specialist surgeon can do this for you, if you—"

"No, that won't be necessary I just need the blood work. Thanks," she interrupted.

She then abruptly ended the call. I turned to Jen and told her Mrs. Jackson would be stopping by for copies of the blood work. Our practice knows that's usually a sign that she is taking them to another vet.

Jen responded, "She can have them! After all your time, that's how you get treated? Ridiculous. You'll be better off if she goes somewhere else. Trust me."

The comment she had made the week before, I had blown off. This time, I was starting to see her point of view.

Second Opinion, Day Twelve

We were wrong. Mrs. Jackson called back and scheduled the surgery. We were convinced she was well on her way to the next practice. Liz told Jen and me that we were too negative. Her theory was that Mrs. Jackson had been scared by her previous vet, that she was just being thorough with us. Jen didn't buy into that theory, and neither did I. We knew there was more to Mrs. Jackson than that. We had the phone calls to prove it. I figured Mrs. Jackson's "people person" skills had done a number on Liz and brainwashed her. I gave up trying to argue.

Second Opinion, Days Thirteen and Fourteen

The surgery went smoothly, and there were no complications. This particular surgery is one of my favorites. It's relatively easy to do, and complications are pretty rare. We sent the three stones to be analyzed and the urine off for culture. After I finished, I called Mrs. Jackson to let her know. The call should have been a simple update, but it wasn't.

"How's my baby?" Mrs. Jackson answered her cell phone.

"Mrs. Jackson, Scarlet is waking up now. Everything went smoothly, and she should do great. We are going to keep her overnight on fluids. We started her on antibiotics to cover her surgery. She'll be going home on amoxicillin—"

"Wait! Why is she on antibiotics? Shouldn't you be waiting for her culture results?"

"After I got her culture, I started the amoxicillin. We have her on antibiotics to cover her surgery and prevent infection. Amoxicillin is also a good choice *if* she does have a urinary tract infection. It's a basic antibiotic and won't interfere with the choices of antibiotics on her results."

"If you say so. Honey, I have given up trying to follow all the details. You're too confusing. I have to run. Can you have the girls call me tonight when they check on her?" She hung up.

Surprisingly, discharging Scarlet the next day was uneventful. Mrs. Jackson kept her eyes squinted and had a look on her face that signaled she was getting ready to ask a question. I showed her the post-op X-rays, with the stones gone and still nothing. I kept waiting for her to spring them on me, but they never came. I even threw myself to the wolves when I said my discharge wrap-up line: "Do you have any questions about anything I've gone over?"

She remained silent, still with a confused look on her face. The silent stare was awkward, and all I could think about was her statement the day before: "I have given up trying to follow the details."

I was rescued when Cassey entered the room with Scarlet. She handed Mrs. Jackson her bag with the medications and the discharge instructions. After she handed her Scarlet's leash, Mrs. Jackson quickly turned and left.

It wasn't until my next appointment that I thought something was missing. She never thanked me. Looking back, I couldn't remember her saying thank you. It seemed, especially after that case, a thank you would be on the agenda. I started replaying the encounter, and it wasn't there. Then again, not everyone joyously thanks me. I dismissed the thought and went into my next appointment.

Second Opinion, Day Thirty-Five

It had been a little over a week since I had seen Mrs. Jackson and Scarlet. I had taken her sutures out, and her incision looked good. We went over the stone analysis, and her culture results were negative (normal is the term I used for Mrs. Jackson). We put Scarlet on a new diet to prevent new stones from forming. She had been doing great, and her urination was back to normal. Mrs. Jackson had no questions for me that day, and she was in a hurry to leave. I got the impression that she was as happy to be done with me as she was with Scarlet's surgery. There was no thank you in that appointment either, if you're keeping score.

 I was surprised to see her on the appointment schedule for a recheck. The appointment said; "Recheck incision. Owner concerned. Lump at the incision area. Painful according to owner."

My mind started racing. Already, I was picturing a huge, nasty abscess on Scarlet's incision. This isn't common, especially this far out from after surgery, even less common on one that we had on antibiotics. If there was one case and one client for this to happen, it would be this one. Small lumps at the incision are a common complication. They are usually mild. They can be localized infection. It doesn't help if a dog decides to lick their incision, hence the reason all surgeries leave with a plastic e-collar.

In some cases, they aren't an infection, and they have to do with the body breaking down the suture material in the layer under the skin. Those "dissolvable" sutures that we use under the skin, don't actually dissolve on their own. The body breaks them down over time. It can take months for them to completely go away. During this process, sometimes extra scar tissue forms that takes time to go away. The appointment was on my mind all morning. At eleven thirty, all my questions were answered. It would become one of the most infamous appointments in the history of my practice.

I walked into the room. Mrs. Jackson picked Scarlet up. She put her on the exam table without waiting for Jen. She lifted Scarlet up by her front legs, exposing her abdominal area, where her incision was. She angrily greeted us with, "Here! Look at it, there is a lump there!" A far cry from her formal introduction when we first met her.

Jen, judging the volatility of Mrs. Jackson, politely said, "Excuse me, Mrs. Jackson. Allow me to hold little Scarlet for you." Jen continued to hold her in the same position. Instantly, I was relieved to see the incision looked 100 percent normal. Scarlet's belly had a faint pink line where the incision was, but her skin was normal. I quickly felt the area and could only feel the normal suture scar under her skin. It couldn't be more normal. I knew the next obstacle would be proving this incision was normal to Mrs. Jackson.

"The incision actually is quite normal. I don't feel any lumps or bumps, just normal scar tissue. Is there a specific area you are concerned with?"

"You're not examining her properly! It is toward the back of her incision. Even the groomer could feel it yesterday." Finally, a second opinion she trusted.

I went back, continued to feel along her incision, and then I found it. It was the first knot of my continuous suture pattern that closed the subcutaneous layer under the skin. It was the size of a large pinhead. Also, completely normal. I had to dig deep with my fingers to feel it, and when I had it between my fingers, Scarlet let out a squeak.

"That's it! You found it! She cried out because it bothers her," Mrs. Jackson exclaimed.

"Is the bump you're referring to the size of a large pinhead?" I asked.

"Yes, that's it. It's bothering Scarlet. What is it? An abscess? I read online that's a common complication."

"No, it's not an abscess. It's my suture knot. Her incision is completely normal. It doesn't look like she's bothering it. Her skin isn't inflamed. Is she licking or chewing that area?"

"No! She is not doing any of that! I said it's bothering her. It's painful. I know it is. You heard her squeal when you touched it. "

"I apologize for that," I said, rubbing Scarlet's head. "It must have been when I was feeling for it. I pinched her skin a little too hard. That wasn't because that area was painful. Look: she has no problem with me pressing on it now," I said, as pressed along her incision. Jen then put her on all four legs but continued to hold her on the table.

"Then why is it bothering her? What is that lump, and how did she get it? You took the sutures out last week. Did you miss one?"

"No, that is from the sutures beneath her skin. We close her abdomen in multiple layers. You are feeling a knot from one of the layers beneath her skin. It will dissolve, but it will take time."

"Doctor, I don't think you are addressing my concerns thoroughly. It seems that you don't like when I ask questions. Do you have a problem when people ask questions?"

It was then that I started to deviate from my usual script. I had been professional up until this point, but now I had lost my patience. Jen instinctively put Scarlet on the floor. She knew the exam portion of the program was finished. That's not all she knew. She knew this wasn't going to be the average appointment either. Instead of her usual stealthy exit, she took a front row seat, leaning against the exam-room wall.

"Mrs. Jackson, I think you know me well enough by now. I have no problems with you asking questions. My time is your time, and it is my job to answer your questions. That's how I am with all my clients. I think your issue is with the answers I'm giving you. You don't believe my answers."

"I agree. I don't think you are correct on this, Doctor. I think she has a problem, and you aren't addressing it," she fired back.

"Mrs. Jackson, I did address it. I examined her incision very thoroughly. I told you it was normal. I also told you what it was, and Scarlet will be OK. It's you that didn't believe—"

"Because what you are telling me isn't correct. You aren't giving me the truth—" She had interrupted me. I had said Mrs. Jackson was best handled in small doses. At that point I had OD'd.

Even though Jen was waiting for something to happen, she told me later she was stunned by what I was about to say. Many times, in our practice, we act out what we should have said in response to a difficult or obnoxious client. What would have been the perfect comeback if we had only thought of it. Sometimes, because of professionalism, we might have thought of the comeback but chose not to use it. This wasn't either one those cases.

"Please. Let me finish. If you are not going to believe my professional opinion on a simple issue like this, then that's a problem for me. That's a trust issue. I don't have a problem with you asking questions, but I *do* have a problem if you don't trust my answers. I have to ask you something that has been bothering me this whole time. I find it hard to believe that you went to a vet for *two* years who failed to resolve Scarlet's urinary issues. This wasn't a problem for you for two years. Then you come to my practice, we diagnose Scarlet's problem in one day—*one day*—do a surgery, and fix her problems completely. In what? Two weeks? Yet I'm the one who you have trust issues with? What's your explanation for that?"

She was speechless. Her confused, awkward stare was in full effect. She was trying to mount a response, but she couldn't. She stammered out, "The incision—"

I cut her off.

"Mrs. Jackson, if you don't trust me this is not the practice for you. It's that simple. I suggest you take your records, and find yourself *yet* another veterinarian. Good luck."

I abruptly turned and walked out. Jen, who was caught off guard, awkwardly followed behind me. I don't know what happened in the exam room after that. I do know Mrs. Jackson sheepishly explained to Liz that she must have upset me somehow, but she was confused by the whole affair. She said she would have her records faxed to her next vet as she made a rapid exit.

Jen, after a long pause, simply said, "I can't believe you said all that. She had it coming. That's for sure. But, man, Dr. Miller, you really let her have it." Jen, like all our staff, had mixed emotions. No one likes to boot a client, even if they have it coming, like Mrs. Jackson. I got the feeling that even Liz, who was Mrs. Jackson's biggest fan, supported that decision. One thing is for sure, I never did get a thank you from Mrs. Jackson.

Mike and Marshall

I like and dislike my clients equally. Well, maybe not second-opinion and holistic clients, those are prejudged for good reason. There are certain clients who actually get special treatment from me. I instinctively go above and beyond for these clients, and they never let me down. I have had clients who we thought for years were good clients, only to be let down by something they did down the road. Whether it's going to another practice without reason or getting into a dispute over something trivial, those individuals turn to the dark side, and it usually doesn't end well. That doesn't happen with this particular group of clients.

I realize I haven't met every individual who proudly belongs to this community. I can say that not just a couple, or a few, but *all* that I have had as clients have been what I consider to be the best clients I have ever had. On a broader scale, I'm not that successful. Let me explain.

As far as the lesbian portion of the community is concerned, I don't make the cut. As much as I would like to have these ladies as clients, they usually don't want me for their vet. My staff and I have tried to figure out this conundrum, and we have failed to solve this one-sided equation. The fact remains; the retention rate and popularity scores with this group are way below average (it sucks).

With gay men, the complete opposite is true. These gentlemen aren't just great clients; for me they are the ideal clients. They never complain, they treat us with respect, they love their pets immensely, and most importantly, they get my sense of humor. If I could find a way to have a practice with only gay men as clients, I probably would. That's why I would tell you that it is no coincidence that Mike and Marshall are truly two of our greatest clients.

Mike and Marshall are an institution in my practice. It seems they are in our practice at least once a month for one thing or another. One reason can be attributed to the number of pets they have. They have three cats and two dogs. They decided it would be cool (it is) that all their pets share their same first initial M. The cats are Milo, Maude, and Missy. The dogs are Mickey and Murray. Murray is probably the other reason we see them so regularly. Murray is their English bulldog.

Bulldogs are awesome dogs. I have never met one I didn't like. In fact, I own one. His name is Newman, after the infamous character from the TV show *Seinfeld*. They are great with kids and other pets, and they are extremely loving and loyal. Lastly, they have a comical personality that seems to be exclusive to their breed.

Now for the bad news. Years of (in)breeding has not done any favors for the English bulldog. They suffer from a laundry list of congenital problems, problems with their eyes, ears, nose, throat, heart, hips, elbows, and skin just to name a few. Unfortunately, skin problems and Florida just don't mix well. Florida is one of the leading states for skin allergies in dogs. You guessed it—bulldogs also have a predisposition for skin allergies. Florida also presents another skin problem for bulldogs. The increased humidity and the numerous skin folds on bulldogs don't do well together either. This leads to chronic skin infections in almost every crack and crevasse you can think of.

When I first met Mike and Marshall seven years ago, they hadn't gotten Murray yet. They had a Great Dane named Marla. They were referred to us by another one of our great clients. You can probably do the math on the particulars of that client on your own. However, I do need to add yet another reason why I hold the gay community in such high regard—great referrals! Marshall had brought Marla in as an emergency. The appointment read, "New client. Referred by Ron Wilson. Drinking and urinating excessively for a week. Didn't eat this a.m. Vomited four times this morning. Lethargic." Just by looking at the appointment, I already had a good idea what was wrong with Marla. If I was right, this wasn't the ideal case to meet a new client on. The appointment was for nine o'clock, and in the spirit of creating a great first impression I was even on time.

9:00 a.m. (seven years ago)

When I walked into the exam room to introduce myself, Marshall Young was standing behind the exam table, and Marla was lying on her side on the floor. Marla, like most all Great Danes, was massive. She took up the majority of the exam-room floor. Marshall was tall and stands at about six four. Even Jen, who loves to remind me, "Everyone is tall compared to you, Dr. Miller," made a comment on his stature when we met him. Marshall was in his early forties. He was well dressed in jeans, a button-down dress shirt, and brown dress shoes, and his brown hair was short and parted to the side.

"You must be Dr. Miller. I'm Marshall Young," he said, extending his hand. As we shook hands, the first of our many appointments had begun.

"That's right, I am *the* Dr. Miller. So tell me about what's going on with Marla," I continued, even though I already knew exactly what was wrong with her. When Liz brought back Mr. Young's (and Mr. Tolbert's) record, it had Marla marked as "Not Spayed." From there Marshall filled me on everything—the drinking, urinating, and four bouts of vomiting. When I asked about her heat cycle, he told me it was roughly a month ago.

Having a dog spayed is usually a foregone conclusion, unless it's pure-bred dog that is being bred. This wasn't one of those. This was a lack of education by their previous vet in South Florida. The five scribbled lines that represented Marla's six-year comprehensive medical history showed how Grandpa practiced medicine. I'd already guessed that they were probably slightly apprehensive about spaying her. It's surgery. We get feedback like that all the time. Grandpa didn't take the five minutes to educate them on why she needed to be spayed. He also passed on discussing the procedure. No, he took the lazy option: "Everything looks great, guys. See you next year!" the result of which was lying on the floor in my exam room.

Marla had a pyometra. After a female dog goes into heat, if enough bacteria are left behind after the cycle is over, it can multiply. If the conditions are right and the immune system doesn't take care of business, those bacteria continue to multiply. They have a party behind a closed cervix, and what's left is essentially a uterus filled with toxic pus. If left untreated, it could have fatal consequences. The risk of all this is basically eliminated when a dog is spayed. Thanks, Grandpa.

Her exam, X-rays, and blood work all confirmed it. Her white-cell count was through the roof at 27,000 (normal is 16,000). On her X-rays, her uterus was massive. It took up the entire back of her abdomen and pushed structures in the forward portion of the abdomen out of its way. Her uterus was angry and filled with pus. On a dog her size, it made it look even more imposing, especially for me. I was the guy who had to take this monster out. Oh yeah, and explain this all to two new clients, one of whom was via a bad cell phone connection.

9:35 a.m.

I walked into the exam room with the X-rays and blood work. Marshall was on his cell phone with Mike, and Marla was standing looking right at me. It was as if she was also anxious to get her results.

"Hold on. Dr. Miller just walked into the room. I am going to put you on speaker phone if that's OK with Dr. Miller."

This happens all the time. I have become used to talking to spouses and relatives this way (or numb to the social impropriety and logistical pain in the ass it presents). What doesn't happen all the time is that I meet a new client this way to discuss an emergency surgery.

"Hey, Mr. Tolbert, it's Dr. Miller. I was just about to go over Marla's results. I don't know if you have been filled in already."

"Yes, Marshall told me that you think it's an infection of the uterus, and she is probably going to need surgery?"

"I had thought that, and the tests confirm it. Her white-cell count is at 27,000, and normally it sits at about 16,000. On her X-rays her uterus is massive," I said as I pointed to the blood work for Marshall. He also had the benefit of seeing the films as I described them for Mike. Upon seeing the films, he interjected, "Mike, you'll have to see this. Her uterus is huge. I can't believe it."

I continued. "The treatment is surgery. Essentially, I will be spaying her, but there are risks and complications that we will be dealing with that separates this from a spay. First, we are dealing with essentially a big bag of pus that could rupture during surgery and increase her risk for a life-threatening infection of her abdomen. Also, her uterus and all the vessels associated with it are very fragile now, and there is an increased risk of bleeding. Lastly, there is always a risk with anesthesia, but with her blood work otherwise being normal, that risk is quite low. Overall barring any complications, her prognosis is good—"

"I'm so sorry to interrupt you, Dr. Miller, but I'm in court today. I'm an attorney actually, and I just stepped out to actually make this call. I should have been back in there two minutes ago. You have come highly recommended. You can give Marshall all the details. I say do the surgery. You agree, right, Marshall?"

"Absolutely. I'll let you go. Call me at the next break, and I'll give the update on how she's doing."

"Thanks, Dr. Miller." And with that Mike hung up, and the conversation returned back to Marshall and me.

Pyometra surgeries can potentially have disastrous consequences. I have been very fortunate that my previous "pyo" surgeries were all straightforward and went on to do well. They had been a lot smaller than Marla, who weighed ninety-eight pounds (that is before we took out the eight pounds of pus and reproductive tissue). That still remains the biggest pyometra our practice has ever seen. It was also the fastest and most pain-free consent to serious surgery we have ever had. Marla had the IV antibiotics, fluids, and overnight hospital stay. She went on to do great, and the surgery went a lot better than I expected for an older large dog.

Jen would be the first to interrupt this story and say, "Don't act like that was so easy, Dr. Miller." She'd go on to say, interrupting again, "That case gave you diarrhea, Dr. Miller." It didn't give me actual diarrhea. Unfortunately, that is an expression that has caught traction among my staff. OK, mainly Jen. She consistently uses it to label someone as stressed out. I honestly do not know how she came up with this expression. My guess is because stressed-out dogs can have IBD just like people. Most commonly she applies this expression when I'm on the phone with a pharmaceutical company or vendor that has let our practice down (screwed us over) from a business standpoint. After I get off the phone from yelling at someone as only a New Yorker can, she'll comment, "You just gave them diarrhea." For added effect, sometimes she'll add a rating, ten being the worst-case scenario for that individual.

Jen would be right. It was a stressful experience. The pressure of that surgery, new clients, and not to mention shifting our busy day around was an ordeal. If I had to score myself on her scale I was at about five; OK, maybe six is more accurate.

Marla did great throughout the entire hospital stay. She was a true gentle giant. We all fell in love with her instantly. As for Mr. Young and Mr. Tolbert, they were more than appreciative. They have more than paid it forward. Currently, I think their referral count sits at eight. I forgot if they sent us chocolate cake or chocolate cupcakes to thank us that time. But I would be fairly certain I ate more than my fair share.

Murray

Marla went on to have a fairly boring medical history, which equates to a healthy life. She made it to ten, which is a solid age for a Great

Dane. I don't want to go into the details on how she left us. But I will let you know she lost her battle with arthritis after medication could no longer help her. Her last appointment involved a final decision, two grown men in tears, and another one doing a horrible job holding back his. Mike and Marshall were understandably devastated.

They had other pets, and they love all their pets like children. But Marla had been extra special. They got her when they'd first gotten together. Since they had Mickey, a three-year-old female black Lab, and three cats, I didn't know if they were going to get another dog. Mike had also made the comment to me, "I don't know what we are going to do when Mickey is older. I am going to be a wreck. I am not getting another dog. It will be bad enough living through this again with Mickey."

Unfortunately, when owners go through something tragic with one pet, they start thinking that they don't want to experience that type of loss again with another one. For most owners, this part of their grieving process is short lived, and they do go on to get another pet. Some owners do not ever change their minds. I couldn't predict which way they both would decide to go, but I was hoping they'd get another pet.

I got the news as I always do, an after-thought from the staff. I'm always the last to know news like this. What makes it worse is it seems like they tell each other this stuff instantly and forget about telling me. Then they'll be talking about it, I'll overhear it, and then they'll act as if they had told me but I forgot.

"I know I told you, Dr. Miller. I told you they got an English bulldog! Remember: you were telling me how they should've spoken to you first since it's from a rescue." That was Liz's response when I heard her talking to Jen about how their (Mike and Marshall's) new dog's name was Murray."

OK, I admit it's *possible* she told me. But she knows how I feel about rescue groups anyway, and she's smart enough to throw that in to make her story that I forgot more believable.

Not all rescue groups are created equal. For the most part, most of them have their hearts in the right place and do good work. Others, however, are less than stellar. They don't thoroughly inform owners about underlying issues with the pet. This leads to owners getting the short end of the rescue stick and ending up with a lot of grief. This could be in the form of serious behavioral issues or lifelong medical issues. That might be OK if they knew what they are getting into, but in most of those cases, owners don't. Mike and Marshall were definitely two clients that I would not want that to happen to.

Well, against my better judgement, Marshall went online and fell in love with a three-year-old bulldog from a rescue in South Florida. They drove down, got him the next day, and the legend of Murray was born. When I first met Murray, it was for a basic exam. They wanted my (late) opinion on whether they'd made the right choice. In reality, aside from gaining medical information about this dog (beloved new family member), this appointment was not going to rescue them.

I knew as well as they did that Murray wasn't getting returned. It was not like a car, especially for them. After that three-hour ride from South Florida, and the first night, Murray was as good as gold. I told all three of them that too.

"Murray, I don't know if you realize it yet, but you hit the jack pot, bro!" I admit it. I was excited that they got a new dog and that it was an English bulldog. I would be welcoming them to the bulldog club with open arms. They would soon find out it was a club whose membership has a lot of maintenance dues and requirements.

When I first met Murray, I was worried. Despite the solid medical records from the vet for the rescue, Murray didn't look too good. The records showed his weight was increasing in his foster home, but he still was grossly underweight at forty-eight pounds (he should have been sixty). His skin and ears were trying to rebound from an infection. His brindle body and white head were peppered with bits of hair missing and scabs. Worse than his skin infection was his zero personality. He was unresponsive and stoic for everything we said or did to him.

It wasn't until three months later that Murray really fully blossomed. I was still worried about his weight, but this time I was lecturing them on letting him get too fat. Murray was now at sixty-eight pounds. Marshall was quick to set me straight. It was all muscle (it wasn't). Marshall also pulled the classic rescue-owner card: "It's all good weight, and you don't remember how skinny he was."

His skin was doing great, even though I knew that would not probably last long. The most dramatic change, however, was his personality. All I had to do was say his name, and he'd run toward me, jump, and try to knock me down. When we left the exam room, he busted through the door and started running around the treatment area, barking and taunting us to catch him. No doubt about it, the real Murray had arrived.

I didn't see Murray until four months later. I expected to see him sooner for his skin or his ears, but this appointment wasn't for those. The appointment read, "Murray Young/Tolbert. Check anal glands. Scooting. Acts like something is wrong with his backside. Agitated per owner."

Anal glands are two small sacs that sit just inside the wall of the rectum. Both dogs and cats have them, but problems rarely occur in cats. The size of them varies on the size of the dog and how full they are. If they have an infection, their size can change dramatically. To give you an example, in a bulldog, they are the size of small grapes. The duct for the glands is small, like the end of a pen. The purpose of these sacs, from a physiological standpoint, isn't known. Not all dogs have problems with them. Whether they get full, or even blocked, is extremely variable. A few dogs seem to end up in our practice monthly to have them expressed; others go a lifetime without a single issue. They are not commonly removed in veterinary medicine unless they become a serious problem, like chronic infections or developing cancer.

So, as awkward as this may sound, in our practice it's a perfectly acceptable appointment. Problems with the anal glands are actually quite common. Believe it or not, expressing them is easy to do, and most groomers can do them. But since that's an area that most people want to avoid, including groomers, that leaves us. We have to express them. If it's just a straightforward expression, then the staff does that appointment. If there is something wrong with them, like an infection, then yours truly steps in.

Mike and Marshall are experienced dog owners. They also have been down this road before and been down it with me. Oh, don't worry. They had known me a while and felt comfortable enough to give me (the straight guy) a hard time about it. At least Marshall did. In the comedy team of Mike and Marshall, Mike is more the deadpan guy, and Marshall is the wise guy. We all (Jen and them) had a big laugh about it. Let's just say, choosing to check Mickey's anal glands in the exam room was probably not the way to go.

Because of that little incident, I was now leery about any appointment in that area with Marshall. I was dreading being the unwilling participant in the Mike and Marshall comedy show. If that wasn't bad enough, I'd be hearing about it again from Jen all day. What I didn't know was that was going to be the least of my problems with them. Things with Murray were about to get awkward, confusing, and frustrating for all us, not to mention this case was one of the most bizarre our practice has ever had.

Murray's Little Dilemma

Tuesday 11:30 a.m.

In the exam room, Mike and Marshall were sitting on the bench. Marshall was wearing jeans, dress shirt, brown dress shoes, and suit jacket. It had been seven years since we'd first met, but he looked the exact same. Saying he ages well would be an understatement. I figured he had the jacket on because he must have been on official real estate business. Mike wasn't working that day, and he was wearing khaki shorts and a T-shirt. He's slightly older than Marshall, roughly in his early fifties. He is close to a foot shorter than Marshall. After all these years, I still can't get over this difference whenever I see them standing next to one another. His receding black hair was combed straight back. I don't know if it was good genetics or the tanning bed, but his skin always looks like he just got back from the beach.

"So, what's been going on with Murray?" After I asked, I felt like the patsy in a comedy show. I was there to set up the pros for the onslaught that was about to follow. Instead of a studio audience, I had Jen, which made matters worse.

I tried to get Liz to come in instead, but Jen wouldn't miss the opportunity to see this show live. She all but pushed Liz out of the way to grab the chart. Then, to add insult to injury, she said, "Come on, Dr. Miller, I'm not checking this one in! You know it all already. Grab your gloves, and *luuube*. It's go-time!" She finished it off with a wink.

"Hey, Dr. Miller. I don't know what's wrong with Murray. He's been constantly scooting. He is getting all agitated about his backside, panting, looking back there, and scooting. I think it's his anal sacs acting up," Marshall answered blankly. I couldn't believe he didn't capitalize on the set up.

I replied instantly, anxious to avoid the comedy show and keep it professional.

"OK, well, let me have a look at him first, and then I'll check those." I did a brief exam, everything was normal, including his skin and ears. It was looking like I might get lucky and dodge the bullet. I executed my escape plan. "We'll take Murray back, get a weight, and then I'll check his anal glands and..."

Normally I wouldn't have paused, but I had been traumatized before, and now I was feeling the pressure of Mike, Marshall, and Jen

135

waiting for what I would say, exactly how I would refer to his rectal exam. "His b-b-backside," I stammered. So close, I thought. I'd just invited the comedy now. Great. Here it comes.

"OK," Mike replied, while Marshall glanced down at his phone. I couldn't believe it. No joke? No innuendo? I started to think I was paranoid, and it was all in my mind. Jen led Murray out of the exam room to the scale in the treatment area, and I exited through the door behind her.

As the door was closing Marshall called out, "Don't forget to be real gentle back there, Dr. Miller." The door closed and I could hear them both laughing.

Murray had gained two more pounds and now was at seventy. I got the gloves and started on the business end of Murray. Jen then whispered (loudly), "You better be gentle, Dr. Miller." It didn't matter, I still considered this one a victory. We both knew I'd gotten off easy.

Murray's anal glands were quite full but not infected. I expressed them. The rest of his exam in that area was completely normal. As I finished, Jen belted, "Don't forget to clean up after yourself, Dr. Miller. If you do 'em, you clean 'em. Don't go leaving it for us to do!"

That's the one last thing about anal glands that I forgot to mention. The material we express is nasty. By *nasty*, I mean words cannot describe the fetid odor of this material. To say it stinks would be paying it a compliment. That's not even the worse part. If even one drop touches you or your clothing, you're finished. Game over. You can clean it all you want to, with whatever product you want. It's not going anywhere. It will be your new worst friend and you'll be smelling it all day.

What Jen was specifically referring to is wiping the dog's backside of any remaining lube, anal gland material, or other fun stuff. In the old days (before they caught on to me), I would quickly remove my exams gloves when I was finished. I would use the lack of gloves as an excuse for being unable to accomplish this final task. Then I'd busily move on to something else, like going to the exam room to talk to clients. Then naturally, as the solid staff that they are, they'd clean up the patient. I don't remember exactly when they caught on and Jen instituted this new policy, but those good ole days are long gone. Now, just so I don't forget, they have gauze pads with scrub waiting for me when I'm done (how thoughtful).

I went back into the exam room with Murray pushing me out the way as he bolted for Mike and Marshall. Jen let go of his leash, and he sat down between them, panting profusely. Jen normally would have left, but she stayed leaning against the wall. She was hoping to get that comedy show she'd missed earlier.

"Everything back there was completely normal. His anal glands were very full, though. Not infected just really full. He should be a lot more comfortable." I quickly deferred to his weight, hoping to close the door on any innuendos. "In other news, Murray is starting to get a little bit more…chubby on us here. He weighed seventy pounds today. He should be in the low sixties. It's March now, and when we head into the summer, that's going to be really important."

I went on to tell them all about bulldog's numerous airway issues and how weight can factor into all that. Just as I finished, Mike joked, "Plus, he needs to get that body ready for the beach."

"Ain't that the truth! Don't we all," Marshall responded, looking up from his phone. "Well, that was enough excitement for one day, right, Mr. Murray? Thanks, Dr. Miller."

With that, they both thanked me and left. After that, I didn't think too much about Murray. Anal glands are pretty routine. I'd solved his problem, and without a comedy show. It was a win-win. That's why I was surprised to see Murray back again two days later.

Thursday 10:00 a.m.

Marshall was "flying solo," as he put it, because Mike was in court. The mood in the exam was completely different from the last visit. Being part of any innuendo-based comedy show was now actually the least of my worries. In fact, I was worried that all the hype I'd made over that had taken me out of my vet game. Because of it, I had rushed through and I'd missed his real problem. I was determined to be even more thorough this time. I started coming up with other reasons why Murray would be "Acting strange. Preoccupied with the back end. Agitated. Panting" as the appointment said.

"We'rrrre back," Marshall jokingly said as soon as I walked in. He was standing, leaning against the wall. He used his phone in his hand like a pointer while he was talking. After I greeted him, he pointed it at Murray's back and started again. "The scooting went away, and he seems better. But something's still not right back there. It's really bizarre. He keeps turning his head and looking back. He looks like he's trying to lick back there but can't reach. What possibly could be bothering him?"

Determined to get to the root of his problem, I asked about everything with Murray. It started to get frustrating because every great question (or problem I came up with) was a dead end. It seemed that with every question I asked, Marshall would have the same response. Any limping? No. Any straining to go? Nope. Any diarrhea or vomiting? None. Any urination issues? No. Is he itchy at all?

"Nope. See, Dr. Miller, that's why this is so weird. Everything is so normal. Could this be all in his head?" Marshall asked, pointing his cell phone at his own head.

"It's possible, but I'd put that at the bottom of my list." That list was starting to get really short. Jen was riding shotgun again. She was anxious to be in this appointment, but this time she wasn't interested in comedy. She was curious as to what was actually wrong with Murray. Join the club.

Murray's exam was completely normal. I checked everything. When I palpated (felt) the back of his abdomen, I squeezed hard to see if it was painful—nothing. His hips and back were also normal. I rechecked his backside again, this time in the exam room. This time Marshall was looking at his phone when he gave the generic client response, "Oh, poor Murray, nobody likes that."

I was running out of ideas. "Well, everything looks normal. It's not clear why he's so focused back there. I'd like to start him on some anti-inflammatories and see if it helps. In this case, they will be as much of test as they are a treatment. If things don't resolve by next week, I'd like to see him back, and maybe we'll take some X-rays of his back." I was hoping for a soft-tissue injury, an injury to a muscle, or some other soft-tissue strain that isn't readily detectable. I was hoping anti-inflammatories and time would save me on this one. Pills and hope weren't going to fix what we found when Murray came back.

Marshall called on Monday. He told Liz that Murray had improved only slightly over the weekend but still seemed focused on his backside, and he was doing a lot of panting. Marshall was convinced that something was wrong. He made a drop-off appointment for Tuesday. Sometimes my frustration starts to get the better of me, especially on cases like Murray's. When things aren't clear cut or they don't respond the way they are supposed to, I start thinking about another possibility. I start thinking that maybe there is nothing really wrong with the pet. Maybe they are being hypochondriacs about the whole thing. They, especially Mike, had never been clients like that. Never.

I have clients who are notorious for overexaggerating. Alternatively, I have others who like to live in denial and downplay their pet's serious illness. Like medical poker, once you know where they sit, it becomes easier to figure out what's going on. I thought I knew exactly where Mike and Marshall sat on this, but maybe I was wrong. It didn't help when Mike made the comment to Liz at drop-off, "I think he's a lot better. Hopefully these X-rays put Marshall and Dr. Miller's mind at ease."

As I'd laid out, my plan was to take X-rays. I'd be looking at his back, hips, and the back portion of his abdomen. It was the last possible stop for Murray. I do better taking X-rays when I know what I'm looking for, and this wasn't one of those. Murray was young and without serious clinical signs. The likelihood of finding advanced arthritis, a back issue, or tumor in his X-rays was unlikely. I agreed with Mike. I thought the X-rays were more to help Marshall feel better than to help diagnose Murray. I wasn't the only one who had reservations about taking X-rays.

If this test was up for a vote, everyone knew immediately where Jen stood. Once she heard about Mike's comment, she wasn't just against taking X-rays on Murray; she was adamantly opposed. Jen thought Murray was perfectly fine. The X-rays were extra work, an unneeded test, and a waste of (her) time.

She felt so strongly she took it upon herself to campaign all morning on the issue. In-between appointments she'd voice her slogans, and make sure I heard her. She'd belt out, "What exactly are we even looking for on these X-rays?" and, "Don't know *why* we have to take X-rays if he's improving." She also used her go-to slogan: "I didn't know we let clients pick whatever tests they want now."

Jen's campaign did little to sway a vote that was already cast. Without further delay, I sedated Murray and we took his X-rays.

As Jen placed his films up on the viewer for me, she muttered in protest, "I hope you're happy. I can already tell you that they are normal." She didn't really know that they were really normal, but she knew the Vegas odds were more than in her favor. At that moment, I would have loved to have busted her and pointed something out, but I couldn't. I reviewed the films, and they were normal. I looked twice, even three times and still nothing. The back half of Murray's body was completely normal. Then I saw *it*.

It was on the very edge of his X-ray, so I almost missed it. Once I saw it, it was obvious. It was on the front of the lateral view (side view) of Murray. It was in the area that represented the back of his stomach, an area that wasn't part of this X-ray study. We caught it by luck. It was radio-dense (bright). All I could see was represented by the outline of something inside his stomach. It was cut off. It was like a bright reverse-C shape that followed along the outline of his stomach.

"Jen!" I immediately called out. "I need more films." She instantly replied from radiology with an answer to a different, more common request. "Those films are fine, Dr. Miller. There is nothing wrong with those, and we aren't retaking them."

"No. Not these films. I need two views further forward. I need his stomach."

Unaware of what I was seeing, she reluctantly replied, "Whatever, Dr. Miller. You aren't going to find anything there either. Let's get this over with, Cassey." Despite her protest, she and Cassey took the next two films.

As she placed the two new films on the viewer, I could see her expression change. It was as if she had seen a ghost. She immediately asked me, "What the hell is that, Dr. Miller?"

In his stomach was a radio-dense object that looked like a perfect figure eight in his side view. On the view with Murray on his back, it looked more like the outline of a distorted hourglass.

"I have no idea, but he ate something. It's crazy. I don't know, but it almost looks like eyeglasses?"

It didn't matter what it was. *It* was going to surgery. I had no idea what Murray had eaten. I did know, beyond any doubt, it had nothing to do with his scooting. It may have contributed to his agitation, but that's a vague sign and a stretch for a foreign body. I knew Marshall would see things differently. Most clients think of the digestive track as a long pipe, which isn't a bad place to start. Where they get confused is on how the plumbing works, especially when it has to do with a foreign object.

When a foreign object gets stuck in the GI tract, the biggest sign that we focus in on is vomiting. We especially get concerned when we see a lot of it. Owners tend to focus on the other end of the equation. They tend to get obsessed with whether or not their pet has defecated. For them, the blockage has blocked stool from coming out. For whatever reason, the vomiting isn't as much of a worry that there is something stuck somewhere. The colon is the widest part of the piping. If something makes it there, that object is home free.

When I called Marshall, I knew he would be surprised at what we'd found, but have no issues with surgery. The hard part of the call was convincing him at what I suspect to this day—that Murray's initial problem was something else that had nothing to do with the foreign body. This current situation, I believed, was the biggest coincidence in the history of our practice. Murray got ahold of whatever this was in the last twenty-four hours, forty-eight tops. It had nothing to do with his obsession over his backside.

Marshall didn't see it that way. It didn't even matter that it was in the stomach. It was the cause of all Murray's problems. When I called him, I explained all about the signs of a foreign object. He even admitted that Murray had only vomited once, and it had been that morning. I started to believe he saw things my way, but he was only pretending. He was agreeing with me only to be polite. He gave himself away when he said, "Mike is in court. Don't worry, I'll explain this all to him. I can't wait to tell him. I was right! There *was* something inside Murray causing all this. I'm not a hypochondriac after all."

As I predicted, Marshall wasn't the least bit worried about the surgery. A lot of that had been due to our long-standing relationship with them. He politely listened and said he understood all the potential complications. But Marshall brushed me off and then said, "As soon as you find out what the heck that is in his stomach, call me. Oh yeah! Let me know when he's awake and OK."

Murray was finally under anesthesia, and the moment of truth had arrived. I had his stomach in my hand. I could feel whatever was in there was firm but not hard. I made my incision over the object. It was quite large, and I had to make a big incision to accommodate it. When I pulled it out, I could immediately tell what it was. It didn't match anyone's guess. It didn't match the X-rays either. Only its shape matched. Like a puzzle, it only made sense only when you saw all the pieces together.

It was a compressed and twisted large thin nylon ball. It was like a baby's ball approximately five inches in diameter. It was deflated and twisted. Its twisted shape represented what we saw on the films. When we told Marshall about the ball after surgery, he immediately knew the exact ball we were talking about. One of their neighbors had given Murray the ball when they'd first got him. They said it had been missing for at least a month. On that phone call, they floated the theory; this ball was sitting in his stomach since it went missing months ago. I was able to dispel that misconception, and they agreed that it happened a lot sooner. Exactly when was still up for debate.

Murray did awesome with the surgery. His backside wasn't a problem again, at least not for anything complicated. When we saw Murray to take his sutures out, Marshall brought us brownies. Liz tried her best to hide them from me. I found them. They were in our microwave in the breakroom. That time when I ate more than my fair share, it was out of spite.

In case you are wondering, we still see the whole gang—Mike, Marshall, and Murray. To this day two things haven't changed. Both Marshall and Mike still think the ball was the cause of "Murray's little dilemma" (as they famously refer to it). I also still have a phobia about that area with them. It didn't help when Murray got an anal gland infection about a year later. The innuendo comedy duo was in full effect that day. We all (Jen and them) had a really good laugh about it.

See You at the Conference

Continuing education is a requirement of being a veterinarian. In vet school, we were told, "Half of what you'll learn will be shown to be either dead wrong or out of date within five years of graduation; the trouble is that nobody can tell you which half." In my twenty-year career, that 50 percent figure has proven to be a bit of exaggeration. The principle holds true that the profession is constantly evolving with newer medications and treatments. In order to stay current, it's imperative to stay up to date by reading journals and going to veterinary conferences. Just in case you're one of these vets who think you are too smart or too busy to go, it's a requirement by your state licensing in order to keep your veterinary license.

I have no problems with continuing education. I have other problems. I am a solo bandito, which makes arranging time off a difficult proposition. I have to depend on the services of a relief vet. A relief vet is a veterinary mercenary. He or she gets paid, by the day, to cover your practice. Not only is it hard to get them when you need them, it's also difficult to find one who fits in with the clients and the staff, not to mention, for some relief vets it seems basic veterinary medicine is open to interpretation. Therefore, not all relief vets are created equal.

It seems as though as soon as our practice finds a good one, he or she moves, becomes a full-time parent, or accepts a permanent position. When the national veterinary conference is on, it makes getting one a near impossibility. They are either all booked, or maybe even going themselves. For this reason, I usually go to the local state conferences, but that year was different. I was going to make an appearance at the big one that's held every year in Orlando.

"Dr. Miller! It will be fine. How long have I been doing this? You act like we haven't had any relief vets in here before. You are starting to give me diarrhea with all your complaining," Jen said, trying her version of reassuring me. It was Friday at four, and I was on my way out. The conference started the next day. I was going to attend until Monday. The conference would go on most of that week, but this way I'd only be out of the office one day. How much stuff could this guy screw up in one day?

Forty-five minutes into my drive, my phone rang. I immediately thought it was my practice, and an emergency had presented itself at the last minute. I barely allowed it to ring and instantly pressed the button on my steering wheel to answer it.

"Hey, Dr. Miller, it's Dr. Jeff White. I just spoke to Liz, and I'm all confirmed for Monday. I wanted to touch base with you in case there were any cases or specific clients you wanted to let me know about."

"Nope. It should hopefully be straightforward and uneventful. I looked at the schedule before I left, and it looked quite reasonable [dead]. Hey, I really appreciate the phone call, though, and thanks for covering me."

"You're welcome, and enjoy the conference!"

What I wanted to say was, enjoy that laidback day, my friend—it will be easy money. You're welcome! Most of my clients don't want to see a relief vet. I'd like to tell you it's because they all love me so much. It's true. I do have a few of those. The real reason is that people don't like change. They also want what they can't have, and I'm in more demand when I'm not available, which means when I got back, they'd all be waiting for me.

Dr. Jeff White was recommended by another practice, more specifically, *the* practice we get along with in our area. By get along, I mean they are professional to us, and their standard of medicine is close to ours. Dr. White had been practicing for four years, and he had just started doing relief. The other practice told us that he wasn't their first choice but quite easily their second, or maybe it was their third. Their first choice was working at their practice for the conference.

146

We have been through many relief vets, and they have all been unpredictable. I have met with some I thought would be great. Instead I was disappointed to hear their personalities, medicine, or both were lacking. So I gave up meeting with them long ago. Jen, in her infinite wisdom, tried to take over the screening job. When her success rate proved to be only marginally better than mine, she threw in the towel. We have since gone by the *Survivor* method (like the TV show). They come for a day. After that, I let the staff decide if they get voted off the island.

By the time I arrived at the hotel front desk, I had forgotten all about that. I was pleased that I had timed my arrival perfectly. I had come between the wave of people that had flown in earlier and the wave of local vets that would arrive later. I stepped up to the front desk, and I was greeted by an energetic middle-aged man. He had red hair, a beard, and thin glasses. His name tag read, "Randy, Cleveland, Ohio." I gave him my name, credit card, and driver's license. Everything seemed to be going smoothly until he gave me my room number: 108. He slid the set of key cards to me.

"Hey, is this room on the ground floor?" I asked as I started sliding the keys back across the counter.

"Yes, sir! It's right down the hall from the elevator bank. Makes things real convenient. You don't have to wait for any elevator. Just get up and go!" he cheerfully replied.

"Randy, I'm not a big fan of being on the ground floor. Do you have anything else, at all, available? Something on another floor?" I asked, fully expecting that I'd be getting another room.

"No, Dr. Miller, I'm sorry. We are all booked up for the convention. That's the only room I have for you. I'm sorry. Maybe something will open up tomorrow. You can check back with us."

I tried arguing, but it was a losing battle. He put the nail in my coffin when he told me, "There weren't any requests for a higher floor on your reservation. I'm sorry."

When it comes to hotels, I hate the ground floor. It's noisy, it feels like you have no privacy, and the view always sucks. If the hotel was an apartment building, I wouldn't live on the ground floor, so why would anyone stay there? I figured I'd make the best of it. I made my way to 108. I tried to console myself that it wasn't a vacation anyways. Just then a family of five stepped off the elevator—a dad, mom, and three little girls. The dad was carrying his swag bag, a canvas bag from one of the drug companies. The family were all wearing shorts and decked out in Disney-themed T-shirts. This was an all-too-common sight at this convention.

These people like to make a vacation out of this whole ordeal. They are usually from the Midwest or up north somewhere. Combining the usually perfect Florida weather and the close proximity of Disney puts them in a perpetual euphoric emotional state. What could be more perfect for a conference than that? I am obviously of a different philosophy. I concede that I live in Florida, and there is a reason for that. I have been spoiled by the weather and have long forgotten the tragedy that is called *winter*.

As for Disney, the New Yorker in me has never been a big fan of what I perceive as one big tourist scam. My wife would tell you that's an understatement. I never found any enchantment in getting ripped off for hour-long wait times, crappy rides, and overpriced tourist food. Like many dads, I've been in the trenches. I tried my best to see it through the eyes of my kids (and wife) and took one for the team. The only magical experience for me was the air-conditioned car ride back home.

I made it to 108 exactly one minute later. I opened the door and received a greeting that reminded me why I didn't want this room in the first place. It was dark outside, but my room was completely lit up from a light outside. Standing on the other side of my window was a heavyset man, with his hair pulled back into a ponytail. He had a Hawaiian shirt tucked into his jeans. He was smoking a cigarette and staring directly into my room as though he was waiting for a show to start. I already pegged this mystery man as a vet. But in case anyone required proof, he had a conference ID badge, labeled "VET," hanging around his neck. I didn't know where he came from, or where he was going, but apparently, my room was located adjacent to a cigarette station.

Without any hesitation, I returned to the front desk. This time I had a brief wait behind several other guests. I made it up to the desk and was greeted by Tim, Atlanta, Georgia. He was wearing a blue suit and red tie. He had black hair that was combed back. I recapped my experience in 108, and without any debate he upgraded me to a room on the seventh floor. I didn't want to be ungrateful, but I had to ask, "Where was this room when I checked in with Randy?"

"It was under another reservation, and that guest hasn't arrived yet, so I moved them. Also, I'm the manager and I have access to certain things that Randy doesn't. Anyway, we want you to have a pleasant stay with us, Dr. Miller. That didn't sound too pleasant." I don't know what guest eventually got into that room, but I have to confess I was hoping it was another vet.

Tim hooked me up with 712. It was a bigger room. Instead of the smoker's lounge, I now had a pool view. Saturday and Sunday were straightforward, as far as conferences go. I hit all the lectures and racked up my continuing-ed credits, attending all the latest, and greatest, hits like "Chronic Diarrhea in Cats: Secretes to Success," "Pancreatitis: Out with the Old and in with the New!" and "Ten Things I Bet You Didn't Know about Allergic Skin Disease."

Since this is a large national convention, they pull in some fairly decent, big-name musical or comedic talent for entertainment. When it comes to the convention, however, I fall into the antisocial category. After the pre-vet club, Edinburgh, and numerous unprofessional medical records, it's safe to say I've been jaded. Most vets (I didn't say all) who I have come across have only further reinforced my own preconceived stereotypes about my colleagues. More specifically, they are people that I would not choose to hang out with of my own volition.

In my defense, I went to school in Britain. Any alumni and professors I remember fondly are all overseas. So when they have all the cute get-togethers and social mixers planned for specific veterinary schools, mine isn't on the program. When Saturday evening rolls around, and after lectures for the day are over, I get another little reminder of this fact. As I make my routine walk of shame down the corridor back to my hotel room, I see all of the assigned ballrooms with veterinary school signs and balloons positioned outside. Smelling the good food and getting glimpses of the party about to happen doesn't help either. Don't shed any tears for me. We both know I'd still be doubling down on room service and an in-room movie regardless of where I went to vet school.

Monday was when all the excitement happened. When I saw the practice schedule Friday, I would have never predicted it. On Monday, I was already starting to think of all the appointments I'd have waiting for me on Tuesday. My only consolation was that I'd have a stress-free day of lectures, away from the practice and not getting any calls. My first mistake on Monday was not adhering to my number-one conference rule: at all costs, *never*, *ever* ride the bus.

This particular convention was spread out over several hotels. Attending lectures at another hotel (the horror) involves riding a big Greyhound-type bus. Aside from the pain in the ass of waiting for the bus and then timing it so you're not late, there is another reason I avoid these buses. My (self) prescribed therapy for this convention involved limited social time. Forced social time with other vets, even for the short duration of that trip, is off limits. Because of these very solid reasons, and since I'm highly efficient (lazy), I pick my hotel based on the lecture schedule. In other words, where can I stay so I can go to all the lectures I want to go to and not have to leave?

On Monday morning, there was a lecture I really wanted to attend: "Surgical GI Cases: What Do *You* Do with This One?" The problem was, it was at the *other* hotel. I decided to throw caution to the wind and go. Everyone has to leave his or her comfort zone once in a while. After I attended "The Hack Is Back! Diagnosing and Treating

That Chronic Cough," there was a coffee break between lectures from nine fifteen to nine fifty-five, which gave me plenty of time to bus on over to the surgery lecture. I even had time to go the bathroom; at least I thought I did.

At nine twenty-three, I was at the bus stop, waiting for the next bus. I had just missed one. To make matters worse, the line for the bus seemed like a mile long. The smart move would have been to consult the conference guide and choose a local lecture at my hotel. I was determined, and looking at the guide, all the other lectures now seemed like disappointments. Finally, at nine forty, I boarded bus number three. The entire bus was wrapped with a giant veterinary pharmaceutical ad. It had a Jack Russell, a cute little girl, and the company's logo and product. Just stepping on a bus covered in a Jack Russell with his tongue hanging out made me feel like I had just crossed over to the other side, a side I had desperately tried to avoid. That was just a taste. I was about to be reminded why I never, *ever* ride the bus.

The bus started to inch away. I heard a loud banging noise from the front of the bus. I immediately knew what it was. A vet had just missed the bus and was pounding on the door. The bus was only partially full, and she had caught a nice driver at the perfect time. He stopped and let her on board. As she got on the bus, I wasn't at all worried about her sitting next to me. There were a lot of empty seats, and I was toward the middle.

The lady was tall and skinny, and I guess she in her midfifties. She had short black hair that was starting to turn gray. She was wearing sunglasses, if you want to call them that. They looked like medically prescribed glasses that were bulky and prohibited any chance of light getting in from every possible angle. She was dressed in a red old-school Mickey Mouse T-shirt, mom jeans, and brand-new white sneakers. Every vet usually carries around one bag. Personally, I avoid the swag and roll with a backpack. This lady had three canvas pharmacy swag bags and two plastic Disney bags. It was as if she was a vet homeless lady who carried all her life's possessions with her. She was also the type of person who is extremely outgoing, but not in a good way. She started greeting random people on the bus, and it was obvious they had no idea who she was. To make matters worse, she narrated her step-by-step trip down the aisle until she arrived at her seat. In a horrific turn of events, she sat down next to me.

"Ahhhh, finally, here I go. Finally, I made it! I'll just sit here if you don't mind. Don't worry. I don't bite," she said, laughing at her own vet joke. She continued, "I am just loving this conference. Are you a vet?"

"Yes," I reluctantly answered, realizing I was in for the longest ten-minute bus ride of my life.

"This is my favorite convention. I go to two, a local one in Michigan and this one. But you can't compare. I just love the weather. Then there is Disney. Oh, my god, Disney! Am I right? I have to confess that's one of the main reasons I come here every year. Don't get me wrong. The lectures here are great, but Disney, I just love it. Where are you from?" she asked me, even though with her inside speaking voice, she could have been asking the driver.

"I live locally, just over an hour from here, depending on the traffic," I replied.

"You live here! I'm so jealous. You and your family must go to Disney like, like all the time! I'm sorry; do you have children?" she asked (announced to the whole bus).

"I do actually. They love it. We never seem to go as much as I would like. You know how it is." It wasn't a lie. If it was up to me, once or twice would have been enough.

"If I lived here, I'd have the annual pass and go at least twice a month. I love shopping there. Your wife must love it. I could go there, just to shop. I'm a big Mickey fan. I buy a new Mickey Christmas ornament every year. I have quite the collection. I started getting *Frozen* ones, the last couple of years, 'cause of my daughter.

She loves *Frozen*. My kids are with Nana this year, so it's just me and my husband."

"Is he a veterinarian?" I asked, diverting her attention from me and avoiding her announcing any more of my personal info to the entire bus.

"Dale? Gosh, no. He's so squeamish. Just hearing about my cases, he goes faint. Dale, he's an accountant. We met at Michigan State during undergrad. The rest is history. He loves Disney too. Now that most of our kids are older, he just finds an excuse to come on down here with me every year. Can you blame him?"

"What does he do while you're at lectures all day?"

"Well, I have to confess." She started talking at her version of whispering, which is normal speaking level for everyone else. "I don't go to the full day of lectures. I get most of my credits from the local conference, and by the time I go to this one, I just need a day's worth or so. Then I'm all caught up. Since I'm a partner in the practice, Dale works it all as write-off anyway."

"Continuing education is a write-off, so that works," I replied.

She didn't immediately answer me back. Then without warning, she started frantically digging through her many bags. She started narrating as she went. "Where could it be. I hope I didn't lose that. I could have sworn it was in this bag. I had it in the last lecture, I'm sure of it."

She paused, defeated, and let out a loud sigh as if she had given up. "I know. Duh!" she said, leaning over into my seat as she reached into her side pants pocket. She produced a big red pen. "Here he is!" she exclaimed to the entire bus. "I thought I lost him. I got him last year, and he still isn't out of ink. Mickey has written up a lot of lecture notes." She held the red pen with Mickey Mouse's image printed on the side. She held it in front of my face, so close that I was worried that if the driver stopped short, it would take my eye out.

She started organizing her bags, preparing for our pending arrival. I thought I had paid my dues and this encounter was finally over. Not only was I wrong, but the question I had been hoping to avoid, she asked. "What lecture are you going to?"

My mind raced. I tried to come up with the perfect street-smart answer that would hide my real intention, confuse her, and allow me to slip away. The best I could come up with was to forget the name of the lecture. Keep the topic, but not give away its title. "It's the abdominal surgery lecture. I forget the exact title," I replied after I could stall no longer.

"You mean, 'Surgical G.I. Cases: What Do *You* Do with This Case?' Is that it?" she asked the entire bus.

"Umm, yes. I think that might be it. I'm not sure of the exact title. I just know what room it's in."

"That's a great idea. I should go to that one. I was going to go, actually. I really thought about it. I am going to stick to my guns, though, and hit "Behavior: It's Tough Being Home Alone." I have been seeing a lot of separation anxiety cases lately. I have a real doozy right now that I am seeing." I was relieved I had caught a break.

As soon as she paused, the bus had come to a stop. We had arrived, and the doors opened. As the other veterinarians and technicians piled out, they all seemed to look back, curious to connect the person to the voice they had heard the entire trip. I may have been imagining it, but a few of them seemed to look at me with pity. One vet who looked at me smiled, taking enjoyment in my obvious suffering. I can't judge, I'd have been laughing too if it hadn't been me.

In what seemed like an eternity, she gathered up her many bags, narrated her way down the aisle and out of the bus. "Here I go. Allow me to step by here. That was easy. Just squeeze through here. Oh, didn't see your foot there."

154

I slowly followed behind her. I made it off the bus. It was nine fifty. I had plenty of time to make it to the next lecture.

Five minutes would have been plenty of time had I made it to the right room. The problem with these conventions is the hotel conference room names. The theme names never match, and then they label some with numbers and others with letters. Finally, rather than locate them in a logical, numerical, or alphabetical fashion, they are scattered all over the place. As I traveled down the hall there was Voyager 1, Voyager 2, Voyager 3, and then Grand Ball Room A. Voyager 4 was on the end of the opposite hallway, next to Stargazer B.

I made it, but I was three minutes late. To make matters worse, the doctor had started five minutes early, pulling the classic "I have a lot to go over so I'm going to start early." The room was packed, and I'm guessing at least two hundred people were there. I spotted a seat ten rows up from the back. No one had the guts to sit there now, because it was in the middle of the row. The vets arriving started to sit on the floor or stood in the back. I'm not the type to sit on the floor, and I'm not shy, so I braved my way down the row. As I made my way down the row, I was greeted with sighs, gasps, and groans as vets moved their belongings to allow me by. By ten o'clock, I was in my seat and taking notes.

About forty minutes through the lecture is when it happened. When I heard it, I was so absorbed in the lecture it didn't register. I had heard it so many times before that for a brief second I thought it was someone else's phone. Its uniqueness was lost on me. The ringtone made it all the way through to "You are going to hear me roar!" It was Katy Perry. I had forgotten to put my phone on vibrate. Luckily the room was big, the lecture was mic'd, and my phone was in my pocket. My embarrassment was minimized but not eliminated. I knew that not only had the entire back of the room heard it, but also, I'm pretty sure they all thought I was a die-hard Katy Perry fan. Several people who recognized it snickered. I immediately hung up the call from my practice, silencing Katy.

I stood up, and made my way to the outside of the row. I was welcomed by the same sighs, gasps, and groans on the way out. The good news, leaving for a phone emergency is not an uncommon occurrence in a lecture. The bad news, as I was leaving, I heard the lecturer say, "And that dog did excellent with that closure. Before I go to the next case, a reminder please do not forget to turn your phone to vibrate."

I made it to the hallway. I called the practice, and Liz answered the phone. Reeling from my embarrassment and having to miss out on the lecture, I was short with her.

"You guys called. What's up?" I asked, without any formal greeting.

"Hey, Dr. Miller, sorry to bother you. It was actually Jen that wanted to talk to you. Hold on. Let me see if I can grab her."

After a brief hold, Jen was on the phone. "Hey, Dr. Miller. I didn't want to bother you but, Mrs. Sweet called. She said Cuddles vomited twice. She's all worried and *has* to come in today. So, she's got an appointment this afternoon at one thirty—"

Still aggravated, I interrupted her. "What's the problem? I know it's Mrs. Sweet, but he should be able to handle that. Is that it?"

"I was just giving you the heads-up on Sweet. If you let me finish, the reason I called is Mr. Burns is here to pick up his insulin. Roger is drinking a little more. He was asking about his insulin. Should he increase it? Or wait until he comes Wednesday when we check the glucose curve? I didn't want your case getting messed with, so you're welcome," she answered, assuming her sassy role.

"Thanks. Have him wait till we do his curve. Continue the same dose. How's it going with Dr. White?"

"You mean Dr. Jeff. He wants everyone to call him Dr. Jeff. I'd say he's OK. So far everything has been pretty straightforward this morning. I did have to steer him in the right direction a couple of times on how we do things. Don't worry, though, Dr. Miller. I can

156

handle it. Enjoy the rest of the conference. We'll be fine." I didn't know if she was trying to reassure me or herself. I did know we were on the same page about one thing.

I am not down with the whole Dr.-First-Name thing. I guess they think it's more endearing to go that way. I'm old school about that. I like keeping it professional and not trying to be everyone's best friend. Furthermore, it's hard enough getting respect from most people as a vet as it is. Throw "Dr. First Name" into the mix, and you open the disrespect door a little wider. It seems almost every jacked-up case we hear about from clients involved a "Dr. First Name." I guess it has its perks, because the clients always refer to it as a positive experience. No matter how bad things went down, they'll say, "It wasn't 'Dr. First Name's' fault. 'Dr. First Name' was the best. Everyone loves good ole 'Dr. First Name.'" However, I do have an exception. Vets who have a last name that's impossible to pronounce, they get a pass.

As I got off the phone, vets were already starting to trickle out of the lectures. There was no point in going back to the surgery lecture now. In fact, I figured it be best to avoid going back into that room altogether. I decided to go back across the hall to Voyager 3 for "Skinny Old Cats' Normal Blood Work. Now What?" I made it all the way through that lecture without interruption.

I got the second bus back. On the side was a giant yellow Labrador with two tennis balls in its mouth along with a huge pet food company logo. As I sat down in my seat, I was hoping to avoid any socializing this trip. The last trip had already set back my (self-prescribed) therapy months, if not years. The bus was starting to fill up. I thought that this one would be crowded since it was the lunch break and people used this time to "travel." A rather large man sat down beside me. I was surprised he chose to squeeze in next to me rather than take the more comfortable option of having two seats to himself.

He had blond hair with a receding hairline. His hair was parted to the side, and it worked well at hiding his bald spot. He was wearing a turquoise short-sleeved, button-down shirt with a tropical fishing scene on the back. He had on khaki cargo shorts and sandals. He had two pharmaceutical canvas swag bags that barely fit in front of his seat. I was relieved to see he had earbuds in. I was hoping he'd provide his own "in-flight" entertainment, unlike my previous seatmate.

As the bus rolled out, he reached down inside his pocket and started his music. It was loud, and I could hear it quite clearly. He was in full-on vacation mode, listening to Jimmy Buffet's "Margaritaville." When we pulled out of the hotel his party really started. He reached into one of his bags and pulled out a two-liter bottle of Coke and a large bag of potato chips. In his process of rapidly consuming these items, I was elbowed a few times. Intermittently, he would softly sing along with Jimmy Buffet. Close to the end of our journey, he placed the remaining Coke and chips back into his bag.

When he elbowed me again, I glanced over to see what he was up to. He now had a perfectly frozen mini ice cream cup that he was eating with a plastic spoon. At first, I was confused on how this item would make it in his bag all morning. I quickly realized he must have just stocked up either in his room or the hotel gift shop. As soon as he finished his ice cream cup, our trip was over. He couldn't have timed it more perfectly. Despite his size, he maneuvered down the aisle like a football player. He beat almost everybody out of the bus, even those who were seated in front of him. In fact, I was still on the bus, brushing off his potato chip crumbs, when he spiked his ice cream cup in the trash and then bolted into the hotel.

I had a feeling that the real end zone for him was the lunch line. This had nothing to do with his passion for food. This vet was no conference amateur. He knew that lunchtime meant one thing: long lines. Usually they had a cafeteria-style lunch in one of the large conference rooms. The choices were limited, the food wasn't great, and it was way overpriced. Without any alternative for lunch, I endured the line and got a turkey-sandwich boxed lunch. The tables they had set up in the room were packed. I took my lunch to a hotel couch outside (which I would have done even if there were seats). I was reading the afternoon lecture line up and in the middle of my oatmeal cookie when the phone vibrated in my pocket.

It was Jen. "Hey, Dr. Miller, I wanted to make sure you'd be available for the next thirty minutes or so. Mrs. Sweet is here. I didn't want to have to pull you out of a lecture and hear you get all cranky again."

She was right about me being cranky in the morning, but I denied it. "I wasn't cranky. I was just in a hurry. You guys always say I'm cranky. Anyway, it's one ten now. That works out perfectly. Next lecture starts at one forty-five. For once, I actually get the benefit of Mrs. Sweet's schedule."

"Oh, that's great. I'm *so* happy for you, Dr. Miller. I had to cram my lunch down my throat. We are supposed to start at one thirty. Thanks for that Mrs. Sweet. Luckily, Dr. White was back from his lunch. She's in the room now with him. I'm sure you'll be hearing from us. Later, Dr. Miller."

It was ten minutes later when I heard back. This time, it was Dr. White. "Dr. Miller, sorry to have to bother you on this one, but Mrs. Sweet insisted I call you. She wanted me to get your input on a treatment plan for Cuddles."

"I'm sorry about that one. The staff tried to get her to hold off until tomorrow morning, but it didn't work. She can be pretty tough sometimes, but she'll usually do what we tell her."

"She was…a bit…difficult. She definitely likes to ask questions. A *lot* of questions. She told me she didn't give her any table food…but…Jen told me about the last time. She agreed on running blood work, and sending out the PSL [test for pancreatitis]. But when I started talking about potentially hospitalizing Cuddles overnight on fluids, she refused. She is quite argumentative."

"Don't worry about it. If it makes you feel any better, that's how she always is. If the blood work is normal, you can give her some subcutaneous fluids and send her home. Have her start on a low-fat diet in the morning. We'll have the PSL back tomorrow, and if she doesn't do well overnight, I can see her in the morning." The plan was simple and foolproof, even on Mrs. Sweet.

I made my way to the other side of the hotel to Beachcomber C for "Anemia Battle Royale: Acute versus Chronic." I sat down, and I was waiting for the lecture to start. A tall, skinny man, with a briefcase sat down next to me. He was wearing a light-tan suit. He had on brown leather cowboy boots, and instead of a regular necktie, he had on a bolo tie. On the clasp was an elaborate design with turquoise stones. I have seen all types of dress codes at the conference, including this one.

At these conferences, the lecturers are usually all in formal business attire. The vets and techs, however, seem to wear whatever they want, and the variability never ceases to amaze me. Personally, I dress like I do at work: business casual. I keep it professional. I could tell this vet was a throwback to when almost everybody was business formal. He was at least in his early sixties. His skin was tan, and it looked tough like leather.

As he sat down, he took off his brown cowboy hat and revealed his white hair that he had combed straight back. He opened his briefcase and took out a yellow pad that was filled with notes. He flipped to a blank page and then asked, "Excuse me, is this the anemia lecture?" He asked in a unique Southern accent that I guessed was from out west.

"Yeah, it is. You're in the right place."

"Hey, thanks, I really appreciate it. These conventions seem to get bigger and bigger every year. I swear, I can never find these lectures anymore, with all the cute names of these rooms. I must be getting old."

"Don't feel bad. I agree. They are all over the place. The names and numbers never make any sense. I feel your pain, man."

He laughed. "Painful, you got that right. Just like that damn bus. I hate that thing. I should tell you what happened this morning—" Just then my phone vibrated. I had to excuse myself from the one conversation I actually wanted to have.

I stepped into the hallway. It was Jen. She was trying to talk quietly. When she informed me she was calling from my office phone, I knew something was going down. "OK. The blood work was all normal. Except it showed that hematocrit [concentration of red blood cells in the circulation] was on the high side of normal. Rather than telling her it was normal and sending her on her way, he started to explain to her why it was on the high side of normal. Now they are having a whole discussion about mild dehydration versus what's normal. Now she is worried about Cuddles getting dehydrated overnight and debating if she should hospitalize her. It's a mess."

"How is Cuddles acting?" I asked her.

"Normal. As in, she almost bit the hell out of Dr. White. I told him to use a muzzle, but he didn't listen. He's lucky. This guy is all over the place. By the way, I'm the one who had to show him she had pancreatitis. Guess who suggested the PSL test to him? That's right—Jen!"

"Well, tell her you spoke to me, and I said she'll be fine. Tell her to take Cuddles home. She can even go ahead and make an appointment for first thing tomorrow morning. That should work."

"OK, Dr. Miller, just remember tomorrow that this was your idea. Don't worry. I'll go and do all the dirty work. I'll talk to Mrs. Sweet. I got this. You know she listens to me. These relief vets should be paying me on the side for all the help I give them."

I went back into the lecture, just in time. Before I could start talking to that vet again, the lecture had started. I kept checking my phone for missed calls or texts. I thought for sure they'd be calling me back. After about thirty minutes, I figured Jen convinced Mrs. Sweet to take Cuddles home. I thought I was free and clear, and I didn't check my phone until the last ten minutes of the lecture. When I checked, there was a text from Jen. "Not an emergency. Call as soon as you can." The last ten minutes, my mind was elsewhere, and I had trouble focusing on the last chronic case of anemia. By the time she finished the lecture, I already had my bag packed, and I fast walked straight to the hallway. In my haste, I inadvertently dissed the formal cowboy vet without talking to him before I left. I called the practice.

Liz answered. "Hey, Dr. Miller. Sorry to bother you again. One of our sprinkler heads is spraying water in the parking lot. I think Mrs. Sweet did it when she backed out. We called the landscaper, and he gave us an irrigation guy. I wanted your permission to call him."

"Yeah, go ahead. If he doesn't bill, I can give him a credit card over the phone. Well, at least Mrs. Sweet left. How bad is it?"

"It's not that bad, but I wouldn't leave it overnight. It would probably flood the parking lot by morning. Uh, um, Mrs. Sweet didn't exactly leave with Cuddles. Dr. Jef—I mean, Dr. White and her decided that we would keep Cuddles here to watch her until we close."

"That's fine. You can text me if you need the credit card."

I knew Mrs. Sweet well enough to know exactly what was going on. Mrs. Sweet had to run some errands, and she didn't want to leave Cuddles at home alone. Almost as important, she didn't want to have to drive home and drop off Cuddles. Letting us watch her was way more efficient. It's also free, which is always a plus for Mrs. Sweet. As long as everything went smoothly, I was happy, even if it was only temporary.

The last two lectures, "Heart Disease: Turning the Beat Around!" and "Thoracic Radiographs: Making Sense Out of Fifty Shades of Grey," went along without any interruption. With five minutes to spare in the last lecture, I got a text from Liz. "Sprinkler is being fixed. Yeah! He said he can bill you."

After the last lecture, I was in in exit mode. I had already checked out in the morning and put my bag in my car. I told you I was efficient. I was on the fast track to leave this conference behind. Despite what I may have led you to believe, I actually like going. In some respects, it is like a minivacation. Unlike a vacation, on the last day I am more than ready to get out, and I am not eager to return again anytime soon. This trip, however, was not complete without one last "gotcha" from my esteemed colleagues.

As I made my way down the long hallway to the parking lot, I passed a young couple holding hands. They couldn't have been more than in their late twenties. If they weren't vet students, they must have been new grads. I hadn't paid attention to make out their ID tags hanging around their neck.

As I approached, the young man, who could pass for Justin Bieber, pointed directly at me. He then exclaimed to his girlfriend and the entire hallway of vets, "That's the Katy Perry guy!" I kept my head down and kept fast walking. I pretended not to be the Katy Perry guy and ignored the laughter. It didn't matter. In thirty seconds, they were gone and I was in the parking lot.

The Lowdown

When I arrived home, I noticed I had missed a text from Jen. She had sent it at five thirty.

"Hey, sir. You don't have to call me. Cuddles did well. She went home. Sprinkler is fixed. Tomorrow morning is full. I will give you the lowdown on Dr. White tomorrow. Have a good night, sir."

You might have thought that text came from someone else. No, it was Jen. When Jen texts, she has an alter ego, and it likes to use "sir." I always give her a hard time on the over-the-top formality of her texts. In spite of her texts, I will try and lure her in to a wisecrack by messing with her via text. To rub it in, I'll start and end them with "ma'am." It never works, and I can never get her to break character. Whenever I confront her on this formality, she always blows me off and tells me it's because she is a true professional. There is some truth to that. But the real reason is she has a paranoia (or

163

compulsion) that something unprofessional she puts in writing or a text will be used against her in the future.

When I arrived at work on Tuesday, it was definitely my version of a Monday. Cuddles was doing great, so Mrs. Sweet cancelled her appointment. The PSL was negative for pancreatitis. When I called Mrs. Sweet to give her the results, it was a long phone call. She told me that I was truly blessed to have such a great staff and that Dr. Jeff was truly a wonderful young doctor. In fact, she said if I ever hired anyone else, he should be at the top of my list. She also informed me that she'd met my wonderful irrigation man, and they'd had quite the conversation. Apparently, they went to the same church. She couldn't believe that someone would run over a sprinkler like that and just leave.

Jen wasn't as impressed with Dr. White. The clients and the other staff all seemed to think he'd done a good job. When I discussed this with Jen, she was quick to clarify. "That's right. They all *think* he's good, because Dr. Jeffey had me. I kept him on the right track. You think Mrs. Sweet would have been so happy if it wasn't for me going into the room after him and cleaning things up. She loves me. I could have a job working with relief vets. That's how good I am."

Every time I mention his name for relief, she insists I find someone else, someone who won't have her do all their work like Dr. Jeffey. She still also reminds me that he left early (5:10 p.m.), and she had to stay late (5:20 p.m.) for Mrs. Sweet. Despite all this, we'll still use Dr. White. He's pretty much our second (or maybe third) choice for relief.

The Telephone Game

As you can tell by now, communication is a crucial part of being a veterinarian. I always thought that one day when I was an old vet I'd have my young buck replacement sitting in my office. I would be sitting at a big desk and I'd ask, "Kid, what do you think the most important tool we have in this job is?"

The young vet sitting in a small chair in front of my desk would meekly answer, "Stethoscope, sir?"

"No, kid! It ain't no stethoscope! It's this right here!" I'd yell back at him in my cranky-ass geriatric vet voice. I'd hold up the receiver of my desk phone and shake it at him to drive home my point. "If you don't know how to use this, and use it well, you might as well quit now!" The point being that effective client communication is an important part of being a successful vet. Giving clients test results, updates, and checking their pet is key. Sometimes, though, despite your best efforts, things can still get all jacked up. Nothing proves my point more than this case.

The Goldbergs were definitely, without a doubt, one of our greatest clients. No matter what needed to be done, they would do. They were friendly and appreciative to all our staff. If you could design the perfect client, it would be them. Except you would want to leave out the next part. Dealing with Goldbergs had one little catch. Well, actually, it could be quite a big catch, depending on how complicated the issue was with their pet. The Goldbergs are like having three separate clients own one pet. Every exam, every recommendation, and every test result had to be relayed to three different people. That could be easy if it's just a normal annual: "Everything looked great today. We'll see him next year." But it could be pretty brutal if the case was complicated and you had to repeat things three times.

The upshot is they are easy to deal with and don't ask a lot of unnecessary questions, but no one likes doing the same exact same job three times. Sometimes, I got lucky, and one of them would relay the message to another Goldberg. Even in those circumstances that only eliminated one person at best, and all the explaining still needed to be repeated at least one more time.

The Goldberg family consisted of Sadie Goldberg, the mom, and her two daughters, Sarah and Debbie. The two sisters were in their early twenties when this took place. Sarah was going to law school, and we rarely saw her. Debbie—I'm not exactly sure what her job was—but we saw her all the time. The father, Howard Goldberg, we never saw. He was like a ghost. I never had to update him on anything.

The only reason I even knew his first name was because it was on the record. Mrs. Goldberg would mention him from time to time. Howie (as she calls him) seemed like a nice enough guy from what I, initially, heard in bits and pieces. Whenever she brought his name up, it was, "Howie loves this dog. Howie said, do whatever Dr. Miller says. Howie wanted me to tell you thanks for everything."

When this all went down, the Goldbergs had recently lost their only dog, Forrest, a few months previously. He'd been a fourteen-year-old black Labrador retriever that had passed away in his sleep. It had been a depressing day in our practice when Mrs. Goldberg had called to let us know. Forrest had been an awesome dog, one that had been like a celebrity in our practice. He had been outgoing and loved everyone he met. We'd seen him all the time for boarding. I'd started seeing him more frequently for arthritis and other miscellaneous problems that older dogs get. He had been one of those dogs that we always thought would live forever. We missed him like he had been one of our own. What made matters worse was we thought we'd lose the Goldbergs too. Without Forrest, we'd thought we might never see them again.

We were all excited when Mrs. Goldberg made the appointment for a miniature schnauzer named Wilson. The first time I saw Wilson was when he was nine weeks old for his first vaccines. Mrs. Goldberg gave me the lowdown on the very first appointment. In fact, it seemed like she crammed it all into one breath.

166

"This is not my dog. I'm just the grandma. This is 100 per cent Debbie's. It's her baby. I'm just the messenger. Anything that goes on you need to talk to her. I have to tell you, though. Sarah is home for the summer, and you would think it belonged to her. She was the one feeding him and walking him all week, especially because Debbie likes to sleep in."

Yes, Mrs. Goldberg likes to talk. A lot. Translation: Call Debbie and Sarah after your exam.

Nine Weeks Old

Mrs. Goldberg was standing in the exam room, anxiously waiting for me. She had tried to play it off as if the dog was not hers, but you could tell instantly she was already attached to Wilson. When I came into the exam room, she had him in her arms like a baby. Mrs. Goldberg was a tiny woman. She had reddish-brown hair that she wore short like a boy's. She had glasses with multicolored frames. She was originally from New Jersey, but the Goldbergs had migrated south years ago. I could still hear an accent, but it wasn't obvious if you weren't listening for it.

That day she was wearing a Boston College Law T-shirt and jeans. I guessed that was most likely Sarah's school. As soon as she saw Cassey and me, she hugged us both. It was as if she hadn't seen us in years, even though it had only been three months. I could tell immediately she was excited about their new dog.

Wilson appeared to look healthy. When I asked if he had been doing well the week they'd had him, Mrs. Goldberg said he was doing great. It was then she spewed out all the ground rules—that it wasn't her dog and I needed to talk to Sarah and Debbie. His fecal test was negative, and I gave him his first vaccinations.

It is hard to predict how a puppy's personality will turn out. Despite genetics, other factors can play a part. Like children, a lot depends on how they are raised. The way they are treated at home factors into their personalities. Having said that, a lot can be learned even at that

167

first appointment. Not all puppies like being handled, having an otoscope in their ears, vaccine stuck under their skin, and the big one—a thermometer in their backside. A dog that tolerates all that, while licking everyone the whole time, it's usually a good sign. Wilson was one of those dogs.

OK, so Mrs. Goldberg was in the exam room, so she's up to date. I called Debbie. She answered the phone, and it sounded as though I woke her up. They weren't kidding about that "likes to sleep in." It was eleven thirty. "Sorry if I disturbed you. It's Dr. Miller."

"Uh, oh, uh, no, you're fine. How's Wilson?" she stammered.

"He's doing great! I think you picked a winner. He seems real sweet."

"Thanks, Dr. Miller, for the update. He is a sweetie. Thanks." With that, she hung up and I guessed went back to sleep.

I called Sarah and got her voice mail. "Hey, it's Sarah. Leave me a message. Later!"

"Hey, it's Dr. Miller, I was just calling to let you know I had a look at Wilson today and he's doing great. Congratulations on the new puppy. If you have any questions call me."

Twelve Weeks Old

The next time we saw Wilson he was still doing great. I asked Mrs. Goldberg about how he was doing at home. "He seems OK to me, but you know this is Debbie's dog. I'm just the taxi service. Sarah had mentioned these episodes he was having. He had one a few weeks ago, when we first got him. I forgot to tell you about. Sarah said she'd call you, 'cause she is the one that saw it. Did she call you?"

"No, I left her a message, but she didn't call me. What happens during these episodes?"

"I haven't really seen what they are talking about. Half the time I think these girls are paranoid. I can't wait to see when they have *real* kids of their own. If they baby them like this dog, those kids are going to be a freaking mess. It looked to me like he was drunk for a few seconds. It was in the morning. No, maybe it was the afternoon. He walked over to his food and ate it. The rest of the day he was fine."

"Did he fall over? Was he unresponsive? Can you describe it?" I asked.

"No, he just stumbled a little like an uncoordinated puppy. Dr. Miller, between you and me, I think this dog is fine. You got two paranoid moms on your hands. What they told me, I'm not seeing. They are all dramatic and describe it like the dog is having a seizure or something. You need to call them. Good luck with that," she jokingly explained.

"I think it would be a good idea to do some blood work today and make sure it's normal," I suggested.

"No. I don't think that is necessary. You know I would tell you to do it if there was a real problem. Why don't you talk to the girls first and see what they tell you. If you still want to do the blood work, let me know. I'll be back in a flash. It's not like I have something *better* to do," she joked again.

I gave Wilson his next vaccine, and she left carrying him under her arm. If you said she should have done that blood work, you'd be right. There was something wrong with Wilson. I was about to find out the hard way exactly what it was.

I called Sarah first this time and got her voice mail, "Hey, it's Sarah, leave a message!" Beep.

"Hey, Sarah, It's Dr. Miller. I saw Wilson today, and I need to talk you about some possible signs—I mean, symptoms—that you might be seeing with him. When you get this message, please call me back at the office. Thank you."

I called Debbie next. It was only ten, and I knew she'd be sleeping, but I wanted to try and get to the bottom of this. "Uh, oh, uh, hello. Who is this again? Oh, Dr. Miller, how's Wilson?" she asked, not even trying to hide the fact that she was sleeping.

"He's fine and I gave him his vaccines today. Your mom mentioned to me that he was having episodes at home. Like falling over or something similar? She said I should talk to you or Sarah about it."

"Falling over? I don't know, Dr. Miller. Sarah has been the one that says she's seeing him act all…weird. She said it's almost like a seizure or something. I have seen him stumble a few times, but I thought that's what all puppies do. I think you need to talk to Sarah. He seems fine to me."

"OK. I left Sarah a voice mail, and if you speak to her, tell her to call me. I told your mom that if you guys think there is something going on, I'd like to do some blood work."

"Blood work? Really? You really think all that's necessary? I'd talk to Sarah. You know my mom. If you tell her to do something, she'll do it."

"OK, Debbie, thanks. I'll let you go. If you speak to Sarah, have her call me."

"I will. Bye, Dr. Miller." She hung up and went back to sleep.

Between appointments, client callbacks, and a complicated cat case, I never called Sarah a second time. I had forgotten all about it until I was at home eating dinner. I thought between all three Goldbergs, if something was really going on they'd let me know.

As soon as I finished my first appointment the next morning, I called Sarah. "Hey, it's Sarah, leave me a message!" Beep.

"Sarah, it's Dr. Miller. I was just checking back with you to talk about Wilson. When you get a chance, call me back. Thanks." The Goldbergs were great clients. But at this point, it was up to them.

As I hung up the phone even Jen said, "Any more phone calls and you'll well be like a…vet version of a stalker who's obsessed with their dog!" She was right. I would have to let the Goldbergs come to me if there was a real problem. They did just that, but not in a way I wanted.

It was eleven thirty when Mrs. Goldberg called and said they were on the way with Wilson: it was an emergency. Less than twenty minutes later, Debbie came running into the practice, crying. She had Wilson cradled in her arms. Liz quickly led Debbie from the waiting area into an exam room. Debbie instinctively took a seat in the exam room. Liz, with Wilson in her arms, continued through the door to the treatment area. Jen and Cassey stopped what they were doing and converged on Wilson. I was writing up a record and ran over to the treatment table to join them.

I quickly examined Wilson. His eyes were rapidly moving back and forth as though he was watching a train go by. His head was bobbing up and down. The rest of his limbs were flailing aimlessly. His gums were pale pink. He was unresponsive and weak. Jen and Cassey worked around me and took a blood sample during my exam. It would take fifteen minutes to have his blood results, but we were able to run his blood glucose (sugar) instantly on our glucometer. A glucometer allows us to check blood sugar levels with one drop of blood. Within seconds its alarm signaled it was done. The small digital screen displayed "50."

Normal blood sugar in dogs is seventy to one hundred forty. Wilson's blood sugar was dangerously low. He was hypoglycemic. His hypoglycemia was responsible for the signs that we were seeing. We immediately gave him four milliliters (roughly a teaspoon) of corn syrup orally. He started to improve within minutes. His eyes stopped moving rapidly, but his head bobbing had now been replaced with a tremor. Cassey started to hand-feed him some puppy food with a tongue depressor. He ate it voraciously, as if he hadn't eaten in days. He was still obviously uncoordinated. In-between bites of food, he aimlessly bit at the air and looked as if he was going to fall over. He was stable enough for me to go talk to the Goldbergs.

I walked into the room to find Mrs. Goldberg rubbing Debbie's back to console her. Mrs. Goldberg had parked the car and joined Debbie after Liz took Wilson back. Debbie was wearing green New Jersey Jets sweatpants, a white T-shirt, and flip-flops. Debbie Goldberg was skinny and quite tall, but sitting next to her mom it wasn't as obvious. Her long brown hair was a mess, and when I first walked in, she was holding her head in her hands. When she heard me come into the exam room, she looked up. The crying had taken its toll, and the mascara she was wearing had started to run.

"What's the matter with Wilson? Is he going to be OK?" Debbie stammered.

"I am waiting for the rest of his blood work, but he is stable. We ran his blood sugar, and it was fifty. That's really low. We gave him corn syrup, and he's already starting to improve. We offered him some food, and he's eating it. Tell me what happened this morning."

Mrs. Goldberg was the one who answered. "He's been fine. He ate this morning, no problem. Then about fifteen minutes ago, he started walking around like he was a drunk. It started getting worse, and then he was on the floor rolling around like he was having a seizure. It was scary. We rushed right over."

"Since we talked yesterday, any other signs?" I asked.

"No," Debbie answered, and Mrs. Goldberg shook her head back and forth, agreeing.

"Any vomiting or diarrhea?" I asked.

"No," Debbie answered again.

"How about his drinking and urinating? Is it excessive?"

"No," Debbie answered again, but this time Mrs. Goldberg added, "Wait. He does urinate a lot. Excessive drinking? It's hard to say; it's not like a *ton* of drinking."

Debbie turned to her mom. "Mom, he's a puppy. His peeing is normal. That's what puppies do."

"It's OK. Don't worry. We'll get a urine test on him later," I said, trying to ward off a mother-daughter argument. "I am going to go back and check on Wilson. I will come back in and go over his blood work as soon as it's done."

Wilson was in a kennel in the treatment area, and I could see him when I left the exam room. I continued to stand and watch him while I was waiting for the blood work results. He was pacing back and forth. His head tremor was barely noticeable, but he was still uncoordinated. Without even seeing his results, I was convinced I knew what was wrong him. We'd had a case almost identical to Wilson a month before. It had been a female Chihuahua named Cora. She had been much worse when she'd come in. Cora had arrived just like Wilson.

Her owner, Mrs. Savage, had run in, carrying Cora in her arms. Unlike Wilson, Cora had been completely unresponsive, and her gums had been white. Her heart rate had been extremely low, and her temperature had been below normal. A lot of owners panic when they see their pets sick. It's understandable when you see your family member experiencing things you can't explain.

Even in pets that are obviously going to be fine, they'll panic and assume the worst possible outcome. They'll run in cradling their pet in their arms, yelling, "It's dying!" Once I rush into the exam room and start performing my exam, I get repetitively asked, "Is it going to die!" If there is more than one family member present, then the question is repeated even more frequently. Despite what most people think, I'm not a veterinary higher power and need more than placing my hand on a pet to answer that definitive question. In the majority of cases that we see, the pet isn't going to die. It usually ends up being a lot less serious than the owner anticipated.

Cora wasn't one of those cases. In Cora's case, Mrs. Savage was fairly accurate when she came in yelling; "She's going to die!" As we worked on her, we all feared she was right. We were convinced she wouldn't make it. We had to give Cora IV fluids and an IV injection of dextrose (sugar). We also had to put her on thermal support to keep her warm. It took a lot longer for her to respond than it did Wilson. She eventually made a complete recovery. When I saw her back for her last set of puppy vaccines a month later, she bit my finger during her exam. That's gratitude for you. Her record now reads, "Use muzzle."

Cora had a disorder known as juvenile hypoglycemia, or hypoglycemia of toy breeds. If these cases aren't treated quickly, they can die from a low blood sugar. When a dog's blood sugar level drops, it can affect their neurological function. Normally, hormones stimulate the breakdown of stored glycogen to supply the brain and other tissues with glucose. In toy breeds, this process may not happen fast enough, and hypoglycemia results. Juvenile hypoglycemia occurs in puppies less than three months of age. Because puppies have not fully developed the ability to regulate blood glucose and have a high requirement for glucose, they are vulnerable. They usually outgrow it by four months of age. The treatment is small, frequent meals. We also have owners keep corn syrup on hand in case of an emergency.

"Hello! I said your blood work is ready!" Jen said, as she waved her hand in front of my face. I had been daydreaming about Cora's case while I stared at Wilson. She then handed me the results. The lab machine agreed closely with the glucometer; his blood sugar was forty-eight. The rest of his blood work was completely normal except for a low total protein. It was five (normal is 5.4–8.2). With everything else being normal, I didn't worry about the low protein. Juvenile hypoglycemia was good news. It's treatable, and it has a good prognosis. I knew it was hypoglycemia. Perfect. Now all I had to do was tell all three Goldbergs. What I didn't know was I was about to give the wrong diagnosis to all three of them.

As soon as I walked into the exam room, Debbie asked, "What did the blood work say? Is he going to be OK?" Debbie had gone to the restroom and come back to looking more like herself. She was standing now, and she towered over Mrs. Goldberg. I'm five seven, and I now found myself looking up in order to talk to her. "Wilson is going to be fine. He has hypoglycemia. It's a syndrome that sometimes happens in toy breed dogs like him."

I explained the syndrome and the treatment. I told them to go to the supermarket and get some corn syrup to have on hand in case of an emergency. After I told them he would grow out of it, they both started to smile. Their relief was obvious. I was wrong, though—he wouldn't grow out it. I'd be wrong again when I told the same thing to the third Goldberg: Sarah.

I continued, "We are going to keep him here today so we can watch him. I'll also try and get a urine sample on him. I will call you later and let you know how he's doing. Then we can set up a discharge time."

"You guys are awesome! Thanks, Dr. Miller." Debbie was elated.

"You guys really are awesome! Thanks, Dr. Miller," Mrs. Goldberg said, doing an impression of her daughter for comedic effect. She then affectionately squeezed Debbie with the arm that she had around her waist. She started back, "I guess we know what the hell Sarah was talking about now. I know you've been trying to get ahold of Sarah, but she's been at the beach the last couple of days. Some help *she* was," she joked. "She should be back this afternoon." Translation: Call Sarah with an update later.

I wrapped it up with the Goldbergs. They left, apologizing to Liz for the dramatic entrance and thanking her for the rapid response. Who does that? Only the Goldbergs would apologize for something like that. They are really that nice. Wilson continued to improve. Within a few hours, all his signs had vanished, and he was back to normal. We continued to feed him small meals throughout the day. I also got a urine sample on him, and it was normal, except for one result. The concentration was on the dilute side. I ignored it, just like I did his low total protein. If I had focused on those two results and connected a few more dots I just might have figured it out.

I called Sarah. "Heeyy, it's Sarah." I almost started to leave a message, until I realized it was actually her. I usually have the opposite happen to me. I'll call a client and get his or her voice mail. They'll have a message that starts, "Hello?" With a really long pause. It sounds exactly like they've answered, so I'll start talking, only to hear, "I'm not available right now."

The only thing worse than that is when I dial the wrong number. I'll start talking to some random person about a pet's results. What makes it worse is the wrong person will even let me finish and *then* correct me. Either way, I feel like an asshole. The staff loves this form of entertainment, and they laugh every time. This time, I finally reached Sarah.

"It's Dr. Miller. Has anyone told you about Wilson?" I asked. I was hoping I could just fill in the gaps, rather than starting from scratch and giving her the play-by-play.

"Yes. Mom told me all about it. I had tried to tell them. That was almost exactly what I was seeing, except it was no way that severe. I know you have been trying to get ahold of me, but I was at the beach. The cell phone service kind of sucks. *So…*I was going to call you today. I feel so bad."

"It's OK. What happened is not your fault. Unfortunately, that's usually how they go down and show up. The important thing is he's doing well now. Hypoglycemia has a really good prognosis."

"What do we have to do now? Just feed him a bunch of times? That was what my mom was saying."

"Yes. I told them every four hours. He can't skip. I'll remind them again this afternoon. Unfortunately, someone will have to get up one time in the middle of the night to feed him. Then first thing in the morning."

"We know *who* isn't doing the morning feeding," she joked, referring to Debbie. She continued. "I guess she can do one late at night. Me or Mom can do the morning one. When do we give him that corn syrup? Mom was kind of confused on that."

"That's only for emergencies, if he starts showing severe neurological signs again. Then you would give him the corn syrup. After he recovers, you would feed him right away."

"Oh, that makes sense. OK, Dr. Miller. Thanks. I have to run. As long as he does OK, you don't have to call me later. I got it. Bye."

He did do OK. Later that afternoon, Mrs. Goldberg left, carrying Wilson in her arms. He left as if he was completely back to normal. I know now he wasn't normal. He was born with a bigger problem than hypoglycemia. All the feedings and corn syrup weren't going to fix it either. In fact, it was only going to make it harder for me to figure out what was really going on. It was just going to help cover up his real problem.

The next morning, I called Mrs. Goldberg to check on Wilson. "Hey, Dr. Miller, good morning, Wilson is doing great! We have been doing the small frequent meals just like you said. Howie said he can even tell a difference."

"That's good news. If anything changes or if you have any questions, call me."

"Don't worry if anything changes, we'll let you know. Thank everyone again for me, you guys are lifesavers. What is it? I'm on the phone with Dr. Miller! OK. I'll tell him! Howie says thanks for bringing his dog back to life. He always has to get involved. Well, I guess we'll see you again for his next vaccines. Have a good day, Dr. Miller."

177

I hung up the phone. By sixteen weeks he'll have outgrown the hypoglycemia, I thought. Except what he really had, he couldn't outgrow.

Thirteen Weeks Old

It had been several days since I had heard from the Goldbergs. There was a message in my box from Liz. "Call Sarah Goldberg. Questions about Wilson." As soon as I read the message, I picked up the phone. "Heeyy, it's Sarah, leave me a message!" Beep.

"Sarah, it's Dr. Miller. I was just returning your call about Wilson. Call me back." It was probably a simple question, so after I left her message, I went on with the rest of my appointments.

It was Mrs. Goldberg who called me the next day. What she described didn't sound that simple. It was around eleven when I picked up the phone.

"Dr. Miller, Wilson has been having the episodes again the last two days. It happened yesterday morning and again this morning. It was worse this morning. I gave him the corn syrup and fed him. He improved but isn't normal. He acts like he's drunk. He's still doing it now. What should we do?"

I told her to come right over, so I could look at him. It didn't make any sense. With the frequent meals, he should be doing great. Even if he had a mild episode, it should resolve once he'd gotten the food on board. She said it happened in the morning. Maybe he was missing the middle of the night feeding?

At eleven twenty-five, Mrs. Goldberg came in with Wilson. Her entrance wasn't dramatic like last week. To the average person, he would have appeared normal. When I came into the exam room, Mrs. Goldberg had allowed him to run around the room. He was slightly uncoordinated but otherwise completely normal.

As soon as I got done examining him, Mrs. Goldberg started apologizing. "Maybe I'm worried over nothing. He looks a lot better now. You probably think I'm one of those weirdo clients that get all freaked out over nothing."

"Don't worry, Mrs. Goldberg. You are not one of *those* clients. Even Cassey will tell you we do actually have a few of those, and you aren't even close."

Cassey, who was squatting on the floor playing with Wilson, agreed. I watched Wilson playing with Cassey. He wasn't normal. He was still uncoordinated. I pointed it out to Mrs. Goldberg. "Wilson still is not one hundred percent normal. He shouldn't be like that once his sugar returns to normal. I'd like to keep Wilson here today and watch him. I might run a couple of blood tests."

"No problem, Dr. Miller. Do whatever. What do you think is wrong with him?" she asked as Cassey brought him back.

"I don't know that anything is wrong with him beyond his hypoglycemia. We'll talk more this afternoon." As she turned to leave, I stopped her and asked, "When did you feed him last?"

"Around seven thirty this morning, after the corn syrup. He ate everything I gave him."

"Who has been feeding him in the middle of the night?"

"Sleeping beauty, Debbie," she joked as she walked out.

After she left, I decided to check a blood sugar. Despite his mild neurologic signs it was completely normal at 135. Just then Liz buzzed back. "Sarah Goldberg is on line one." It was if she knew we just got his blood sugar. It was more likely that she just got off the phone with Mrs. Goldberg. I picked up the phone.

"Hey, Dr. Miller, I think you see why I called you yesterday. I wasn't there this morning, but I saw the episode yesterday. I can tell you my mom isn't overreacting."

"It's OK. I believe her." I was wondering if, despite our conversation, Mrs. Goldberg was still worried we thought she was crazy when she spoke to Sarah.

"Dr. Miller, between you and me, if Debbie missed a feeding, could that be causing all this? I just got off the phone with Mom, and she was worried that…that Debbie might not have fed him in the middle of the night."

"It's possible, but it's probably not that. Usually with hypoglycemia the signs resolve once he eats. He still looks uncoordinated. I am going to watch him. We'll see how he does. I might do more blood work. I'll know more later."

"OK, Dr. Miller. Keep me posted. Bye."

I had just avoided discussing a test I was about to run on Wilson with both Goldbergs. Hear me out. I had a good reason for leaving the Goldbergs in the dark. I had only just thought of the test when Cassey was on the floor playing with Wilson. It wasn't until later that I figured out how I was going to pull it off. It's the bile acids test, the complicated one from that second-opinion case. It was even more complicated running it on Wilson.

Normally, we run it on fasted dogs. Wilson wouldn't do well holding his food for twelve hours. He'd have an episode. I had to figure out how I could do a fasting blood test on a dog that can't be fasted. I wasn't about to start talking about all of that with three Goldbergs. Normally we also get official consent before running a test (we aren't one of those types of practices). This was the Goldberg's, and it was a blood sample. This particular test has to get sent out to the outside lab. So if they wanted to decline the test, we wouldn't send it.

He was fed at seven thirty, and I was going to skip his afternoon meal. If he made it, I would do the bile acids test later with an eight-hour fast. If he started to have an episode, then we would pull blood right then. That would be part one of his bile acids test.

Wilson didn't last until the three-thirty fasted blood sample. At around 1:00 p.m., Jen called out, "Dr. Miller!" I ran from my office to the treatment area. Wilson was in a cage, lying on his side and paddling his legs. He eyes were rapidly moving back and forth, and he was thrashing side to side. Jen immediately scooped him up, and we converged at the treatment table. I drew the first part of the bile acids test. I also checked another blood sugar: ninety. It was looking like this wasn't hypoglycemia. As soon as Jen and I got his blood, I gave him four milliliters of corn syrup. Jen then hand-fed him. Like all the previous episodes, he recovered in twenty minutes.

Two hours later, we pulled the second part of his test. It was just after three o'clock. I called Mrs. Goldberg. It was time to fill them in. "Hey, it's Dr. Miller. Wilson is doing fine. You definitely weren't freaked out over nothing. I don't think he has hypoglycemia."

"Well, what could it be then? What you told us made perfect sense. What else would cause the low blood sugar?"

"I did another test on his liver. It tests liver function. It's called a bile acid test. He might have a liver shunt." I then told her everything. I formally got her permission to send the blood to the lab, all about the test, and what a liver shunt is. I explained that in a shunt, the liver doesn't filter Wilson's blood. His blood still has another pathway around the liver. Because of this, his liver might not be storing and metabolizing sugar properly.

"Is it treatable?" she asked.

"Yes. The treatment is surgery. The surgery is done at a local specialist hospital. The prognosis depends on the nature of the shunt. If the shunt is simple, then the prognosis is very good. The surgery will cure it. But we need to wait for the test results. I should have them in the morning. Then we'll talk more."

"OK, Dr. Miller. Please call the girls. There is no way I could explain all that to them. I'm sure they are going to have a lot of questions. I'll talk to Howie. He's so laidback about the whole thing. I swear that man never worries about anything. I'll let you go, Dr.

Miller." One Goldberg down, two to go. Well, if you're counting Howie (I never do), then it's two down.

I called Sarah next. I was expecting to get her voice mail and get out of explaining it to her until morning. No luck. I went through all that a second time. Debbie answered her phone as well, and that made three times with three complicated explanations. Debbie's call was the worst of the three because she started to cry toward the end. She tried to hide it, so I played along that everything was OK, instead of pointing it out by trying to console her.

After I got off the phone with Debbie, I hoped I was right. If it wasn't a shunt, then it might be something a lot worse, something that potentially wasn't treatable. The next things on the list would be neurologic conditions. That would be a different story entirely. Conditions way beyond my "inch-deep" neurology knowledge. But even my inch of knowledge knew the prognosis for any of those wouldn't be good. Going through that with the Goldbergs would be devastating.

The next morning the bile acids test came back. I made my fast walk to my box, where the staff puts the records with blood work results, for Wilson's chart. I opened it, and the lab results were sitting right on top.

Goldberg, Wilson

Pre-Meal Bile Acids: 127.5 (normal less than 10)

Post-Meal Bile Acids: 129.4 (normal less than 20)

They were through the roof, conclusive for a portosystemic shunt (liver shunt). It all made sense, especially the low-normal protein and dilute urine that I'd overlooked. I felt I'd let the Goldbergs down. I started thinking that maybe I should have picked up on it earlier. The truth is that's how some cases play out. They aren't always obvious from the start.

I called all three Goldbergs, I didn't get lucky with Sarah either. She picked up on the second ring. One by one, I told them that Wilson had a shunt. I also told them all again; the treatment was surgery, and the prognosis all depended on the type of shunt.

The good news was the specialist was always an option for the Goldbergs. Mrs. Goldberg had put me on hold after I told her about surgery. Even though she knew, as well as I did, it was a foregone conclusion. She went through the standard Goldberg protocol anyway and asked Howie. When she came back on the phone she said, "Howie says to do whatever *you* say to do. Call the specialist. We'll do the surgery."

Fourteen Weeks Old (Monday)

The Goldbergs went to the specialists. They confirmed that Wilson had a portosystemic shunt. They did the surgery. The shunt was simple, and his prognosis was excellent. They kept him for two days and then sent him home. After we sent him to the specialists, we got two sets of updates for everything, one call from the specialists and another one from Mrs. Goldberg. I was surprised that the Goldbergs never called once he'd gotten home. I was beginning to worry that something happened. I finally heard back from them on Monday. They reached out in a way that caught us all by surprise.

I just came out of the room with Mrs. Sweet and Cuddles. It's a long story. I'll try and keep it short, but it's Mrs. Sweet and nothing is ever short with her. She was back for a recheck on a scratch on Cuddles's left eye (corneal ulcer). I had explained to her several times that blindness wasn't an outcome for this type of injury. It didn't matter. She was obsessed from the start that the small scratch would somehow make Cuddles blind. It had healed. She was so relieved that Cuddles wouldn't be going blind that she went into full-on *sweet* mode. There might have been a hug involved, but don't quote me on that.

In case you wanted to know about wardrobe, Mrs. Sweet was still feeling the Fourth of July spirit. She was wearing a white T-shirt with a black poodle on it. The poodle was wearing a bedazzled red, white, and blue top hat. On the bottom, in red bedazzled letters, it said, "Independence Day 1776." I guess it didn't bother her that it was September.

As soon as I walked out I could see it. I saw it even before Jen said: "Look what we got. At least someone appreciates us girls—and we know it's not you!" It was one of those edible fruit arrangements, probably one of the largest I have even seen. It had cantaloupes, melons, pineapples, and strawberries. Some of the strawberries were covered in chocolate. Attached was a Mylar balloon that said, "THANK YOU!"

It was from the Goldbergs. Sarah had dropped it off when I was in the exam room. Along with it was a thank-you card: "To Dr. Miller and all the girls, thank you so much for taking care of Wilson. He is doing awesome! You guys are the best! The Goldbergs."

I hadn't even finished reading it, when Jen said, "Don't start eating it all, Dr. Miller. We know how you are. Save some for us! We are the ones that do all the work. All you do is talk on the phone. I hope they got the specialists one of these. They did all the real work on that case." She joked, even though it didn't really sound like one, especially the part about me eating it all. I barely touched it. OK, by now you know, I ate more than my fair share. This time it was because, despite what Jen thought, I deserved it!

I have to admit, overall, it was a good day, especially for a Monday. Yeah, yeah, I know what I said about Mondays. That's still true. Trust me: it is. Consider that Monday a freak occurrence. An exception to my saying that nobody wants to be a vet on Monday. That particular Monday maybe someone actually wanted to be a vet. That's all you'll get out of me. This isn't one of those touchy-feely books.

Let's face it—you knew this whole good-day thing, it wouldn't last long. The next day was classic and not in a good way either. The case that I saw on Tuesday, that was an entirely different story.

184

There was no balloon, card, or fruity chocolate at the end of that one. That client was definitely no Goldberg.

When I talked to Jen about that case being the next chapter, she was quick to offer her advice: "The book is fine, Dr. Miller! How much are you going to write? You don't pay us enough to do all this proofreading. If I have to read about the Tuesday client, after just living through it, I'm the one who is going to have diarrhea!"

I figured I'd take her advice.

At least this time.

what does a pirate tell
you when you ask what his
age is, the day ~~after his birthday~~ he is
an octo-
genarian

aye, matey

CPSIA information can be obtained
at www.ICGtesting.com
Printed in the USA
BVHW031927010520
579060BV00002B/445

9 780692 902806